COSMOPOLITAN
SEX
OPE
DIA

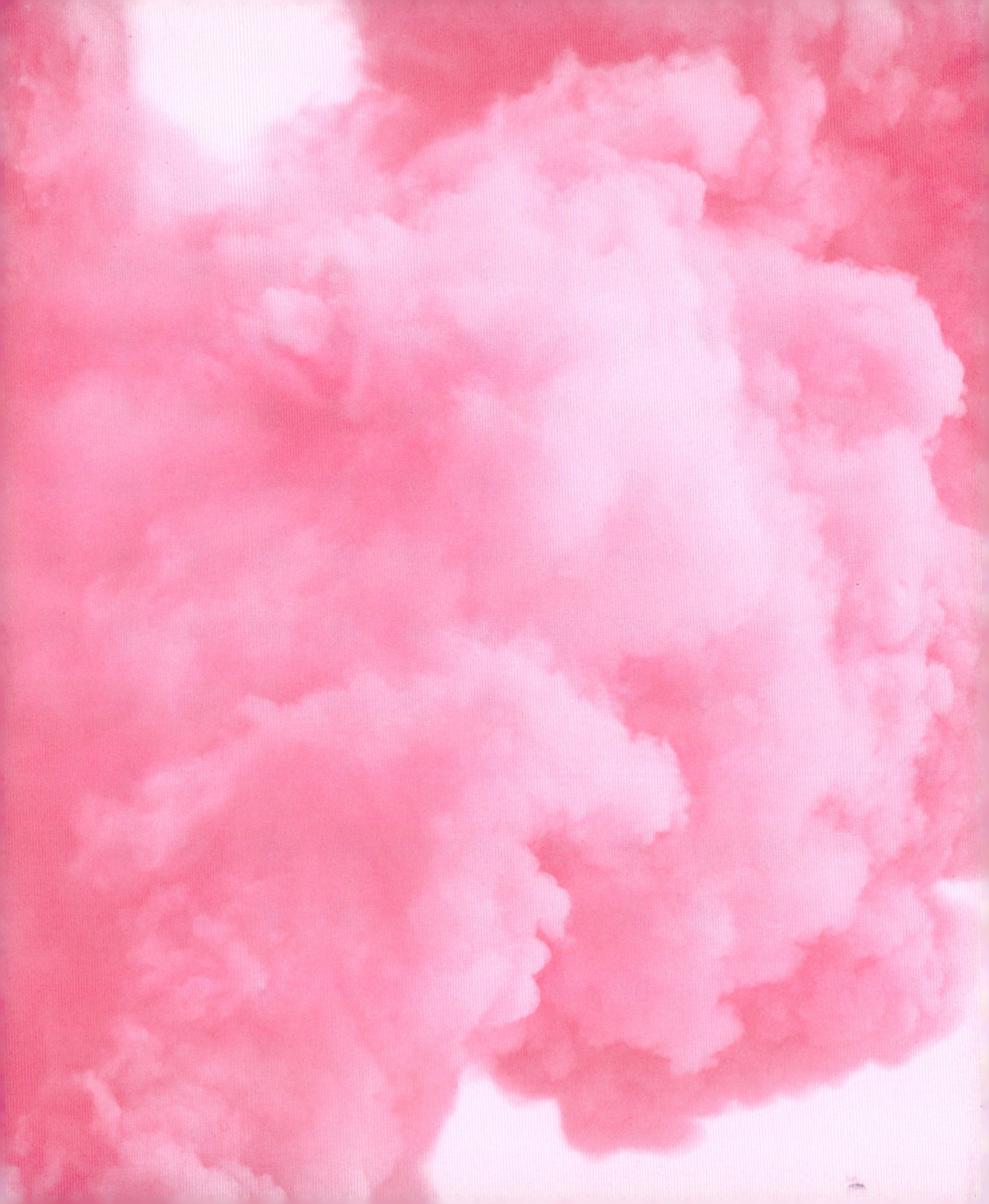

COSMOPOLITAN

SEXOPEDIA

Your Ultimate A to Z Guide to Getting it On

HEARST
books

A B C D E F G

10
Allorgasmia
Amorous
Anal
Anal Bleaching
Anal Play
Androsexuality
Anorgasmia
Asexuality
Autofellatio

20
Balls
Bareback
BDSM
Bisexuality
Blow Job
Blue Balls
Breasts
Boobgasm
Butt Plug

34
Circumcision
Cisgender
Clitoris
Condoms
Consensual Nonmonogamy
Consent
Coregasm
Cosplay
Creampie
Cum
Cum Shot
Cunnilingus

48
Deep Throating
Dicktionary
Dildo
DILF
Dirty Talk
Doggy Style
Double Penetration
Dry Orgasm
DTF

56
Edging
Ejaculation
Erection
Erotica
Erotophilic
Erotophobic
Eunuch

62
Facial
Fellatio
Fetish
Fingering
Fisting
Foot Job
Foreplay
Fourchette
Fuck

72
G-Spot
Gay
Gender
Genderqueer
Genitalia
GNOC
Golden Shower

N O P Q R S

122
Naturist
Nipples
Nipple Clamps
Nonbinary
NSFW

128
Oral Sex
Orgasm
Orgy

138
Pansexuality
Pearl Necklace
Pegging
Penis
Piercings
PNV
Polyamory
Pompoir
Positions
Precum
Pubic Hair

156
Queefing
Queening
Queer
Quickie

162
Refractory Period
Reverse Cowgirl
Rimming
Rough Sex
Rusty Trombone

170
Safe Word
Scissoring
Semen
Sext
Sex Toys
Sexual Intercourse
Shower Sex
Sixty-Nine
Squirting
Sugarpic
STI

H I J K L M

78
Hair Removal
Hand Job
Happy Ending
Hard-On
Heterosexuality/
Homosexuality
Horny

84
Impotence
Incest
Intersex
Ithyphallophobia

90
Jelqing
Jerking Off

94
Kama Sutra
Kegels
Kink
Kissing
KOTL

102
Labia
Lesbian
Lesbian Sex
Libido
Lube

112
M-Zone
Masochist
Masturbation
Mile-High Club
MILF
Missionary
Money Shot
Monogamy
Morning-After Pill
Morning Wood
Motorboating

T U V W X Y Z

190
Tantric Sex
TDTM
Teabagging
Threesome
Tit Fucking
Tossed Salad
Transgender
Tune in Tokyo

202
Uncircumcised

204
Vagina
VCH Piercing
Vibrator
Virgin
Vulva

212
Wank
Watersports
Wet Dreams
Withdrawal
WSN

216
X-Rated

218
Yes Means Yes

220
Z-Job
Zelophobia

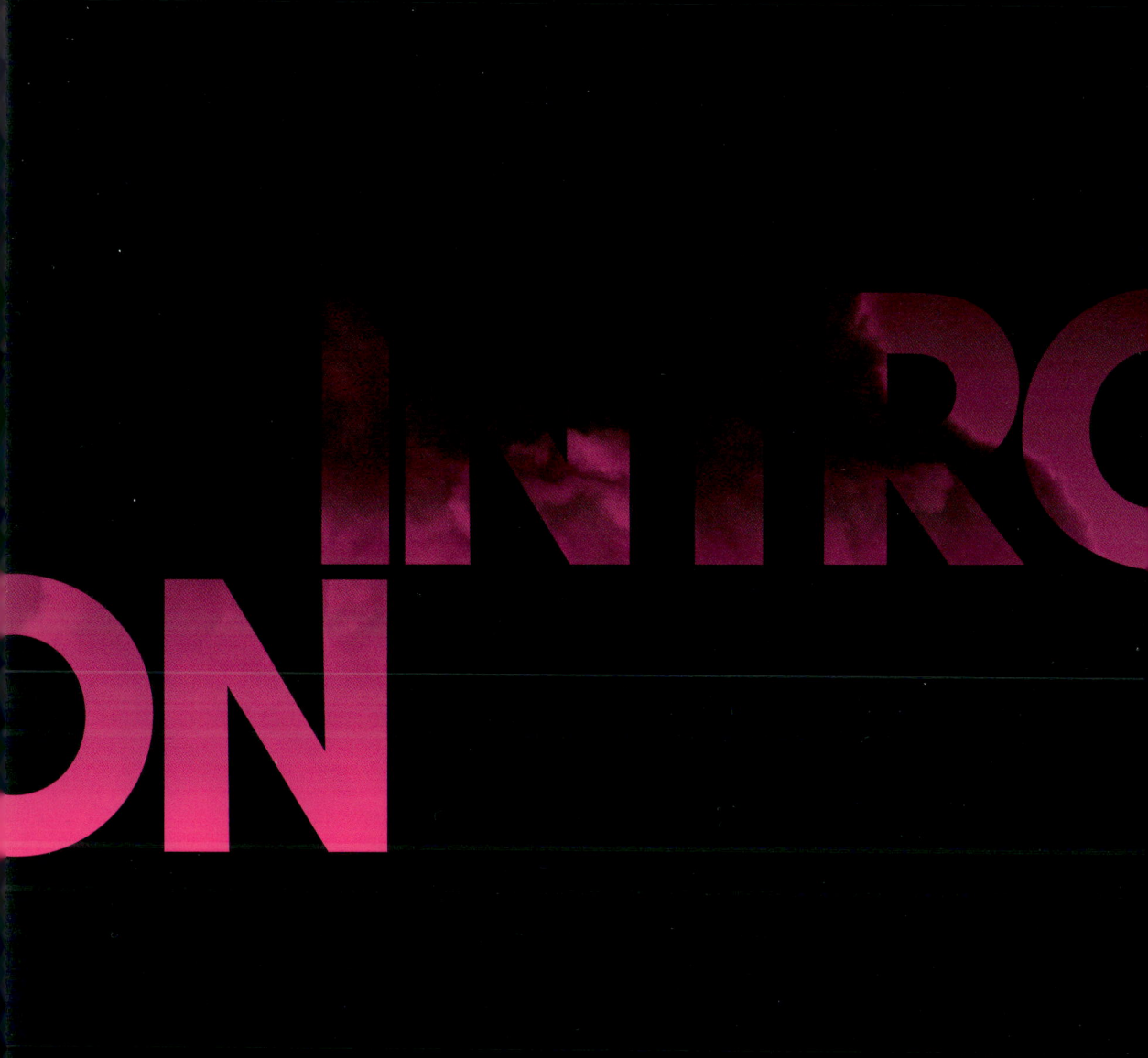

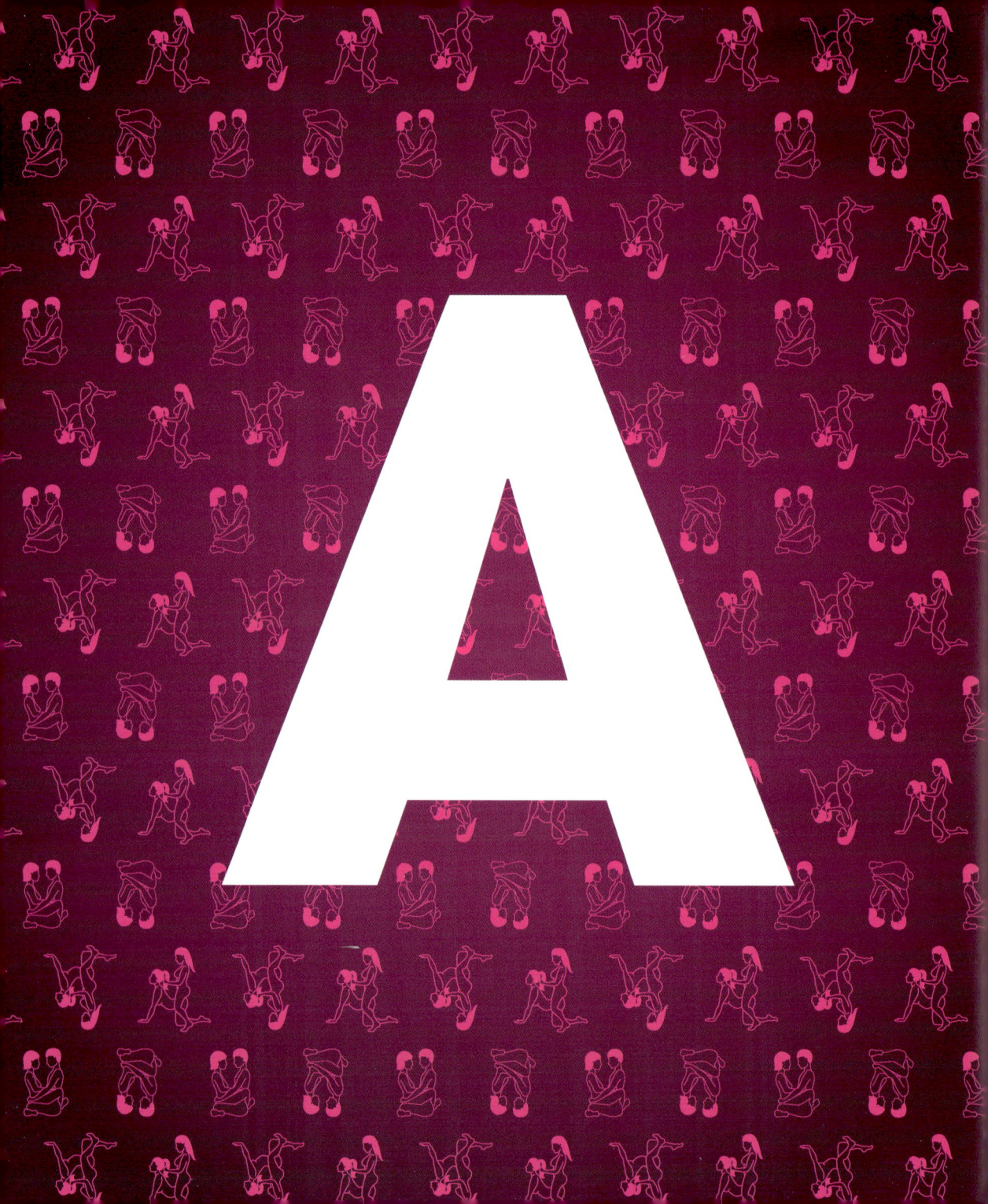

allorgasmia

An oddly scary-sounding name for a really NBD thing. Allorgasmia happens when you're having sex with your significant other but find yourself fantasizing about someone else (ahhh, Ryan Gosling) in order to get off. This doesn't mean you like your mate any less, says sexologist Emily Morse, host of the podcast *Sex with Emily*. "Think about it like this: You aren't replacing your physical connection with your partner. You're enhancing it by tapping into your fantasies." If it's not leading to obsession, anxiety, or reactions that could hurt your relationship, says Morse, then let your mind run wild.

RELATED TERMS:
anorgasmia, erotophilic/ erotophobic, ithyphallophobia, zelophobia

---

amorous

That super hot-and-sensual feeling you get when all your senses are hyper-focused on sexual desire and love. But here are some fun stuff that you may not know:

- **Men who are turned on smell different**—at least to the subconscious. According to research at Rice University, when women smelled sweat created by a man watching porn, a different part of their brains lit up than when they smelled normal workout sweat. This research supports the idea that our brains may be processing chemical signals from other humans in ways we aren't always aware of.

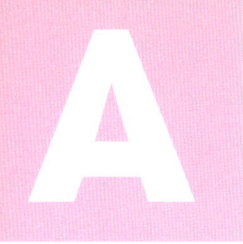

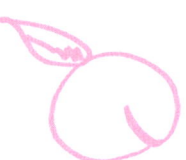

- **Some people sneeze when feeling revved up,** reports a study in the *Journal of the Royal Society of Medicine*. The reason? Mixed-up signals in the body. The parasympathetic nervous system—which helps you get ready for sex by sparking lubrication or clitoral arousal—can also accidentally cause fluid to flow in the nose, making a person sneeze. (These crossed signals may also be the reason why bright lights make some people *achoo*.)

- **The peak time of day women desire sex is 11:21 p.m.** while for men, it's 7:54 a.m.—at least according to a survey by sex-toy company Lovehoney®.

- **And, apparently, men are more sexually attracted to women's bare bodies in the winter** than in the summer, according to research by Dr. Justin Lehmiller. Because there tends to be less flesh on display, seeing skin in January is more novel and arousing.

✺ **RELATED TERMS:**
libido, horny

anal

General interest in backdoor love is definitely trending up, with sex experts saying it's the move that women ask them about most. In fact, 35.9 percent of heterosexual women and 42.3 percent of heterosexual men ages 18–44 in the US have tried it.

Anal sex is typically thought of as anal penetration with a penis. And while pleasure can't be boiled down to just one thing, there are aspects of anal sex that both men and women can enjoy. Some guys like going *there* with a woman because the anus is tighter than the vagina, giving his D a more intense feeling during intercourse. Some women find that because of the rich cluster of nerves surrounding the anus, the area is a powerful zone.

According to Dr. Kat Van Kirk, a clinical sexologist and marriage-and-family therapist, these are four of the most common misconceptions about anal sex:

MYTH #1: It's going to hurt.
Anal sex doesn't have to be painful; it's often just done incorrectly. Many women find it incredibly pleasurable, and some even report having orgasms. If you and your partner start slowly—using fingers and smaller sex toys with plenty of lube, pain will be the last thing on your mind. If you've had a bad experience, it doesn't mean you shouldn't try it again. Most painful experiences have to do with not following the above instructions. Plus, here's a trick to help you relax: Stimulate your clitoris at the same time during anal and it can encourage the pleasure-over-pain response.

MYTH #2: It's dirty (and not in a sexy way).
The anus and lower part of the rectum actually have very little fecal material. You do, however, need to be careful about transferring anything from the anus into the vagina, as even microscopic elements can cause vaginal infections. So consider having anal at the end of your session.

MYTH #3: It can physically damage you.
Well, having any sort of sex the "wrong way" could cause damage. Think about it: If you're vaginally dry and don't use additional lube, you can cause micro-tears in the vagina. The same thing can happen in anal sex. Granted, the anus doesn't create its own lubrication like the vagina does, but that just means real lube (not saliva, which dries quickly) needs to be used for a healthy experience.

MYTH #4: You don't need to use condoms.
Some people assume that because there's no pregnancy risk, they don't need to use a condom. WRONG. Most STIs are transferrable through the anus (including chlamydia, gonorrhea, infectious hepatitis, and HIV), because the lining of the anus is thinner and can be broken more easily if too much dry friction occurs (again, remember, to lube up).

MYTH
In a study published in the *Journal of Sexual Medicine*, less than 40 percent of gay men surveyed engaged in anal intercourse during their last sexual event. What was the most popular answer? Kissing.

⭐ **RELATED TERMS:**
anal bleaching, anal play, butt plug, double penetration, lube, pegging, rimming, rusty trombone, STI, tossed salad

anal play

This refers to other types of backdoor action that don't involve a penis.

- **Anal toys:** A variety of items intended for anal sex, including anal beads (a string of round beads that are often inserted one by one and then pulled out) and butt plugs (which typically have a tapered shape that flares at the bottom).

- **Fisting:** When a partner inserts a fist in the other partner's rectum. Fisting, also called *handballing*, can be used for vaginal stimulation as well.

- **Pegging:** When a woman performs anal intercourse on a man with the help of a strap-on dildo. A woman can also peg another woman.

- **Rimming:** Licking, sucking, and pleasuring a partner's anus with lips, tongue, and mouth. Also called *rim job*, *tossed salad*, and *anilingus*.

RELATED TERMS:
anal, butt plug, pegging, rimming, rusty trombone, tossed salad

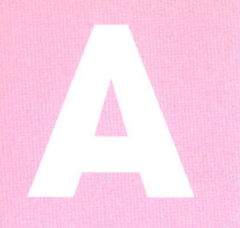

> "THE MOST COMMON DEFINITION OF *ANDROSEXUAL* IS A PERSON WHO IS ATTRACTED TO INDIVIDUALS ON THE MASCULINE SIDE OF THE GENDER SPECTRUM."

androsexuality

There are a few meanings of the term *androsexual* says Dr. Jay Irwin, associate professor of sociology at the University of Nebraska at Omaha. "The most common definition of *androsexual* is a person who is attracted to individuals on the masculine side of the gender spectrum. Sometimes this is interpreted as individuals who are attracted to cisgender men (that is, people who were assigned male at birth and also identify as a man), but that binary-based definition is typically too narrow for how individuals who identify as androsexual see their sexuality."

It is possible that a person who identifies as androsexual might be attracted to someone assigned as female at birth but who has a more masculine vibe. Finally, a less commonly used definition of *androsexual* refers to people who feel sexual attraction to gender neutral or non-gendered individuals.

RELATED TERMS:
asexuality, bisexuality, cisgender, gay, gender, genderqueer, heterosexuality/ homosexuality, lesbian, nonbinary, pansexuality, transgender, queer

anorgasmia

Perhaps one of the suckiest words in this entire book, *anorgasmia* describes the inability to have an orgasm. It can happen to both sexes, but according to the Global Library of Women's Medicine, it's much more common in women. In one study, 24 percent of the women surveyed reported orgasmic dysfunction. Causes include medication, drugs or alcohol, anxiety or other psychological factors, gynecological issues, and hormonal changes.

If you find yourself in a no-orgasm-for-you-ever situation, talk with your gynecologist or other medical professionals to rule out health issues first. Then you might want to start playing around with all your pleasure spots. Remember that a vast majority of women require clitoral stimulation—not just vaginal penetration—to orgasm, so it's very possible that you haven't tried what works for you yet.

According to James Kashanian, MD, a urologist at New York–Presbyterian Hospital Cornell, there are a few different ways that anorgasmia manifests in men. There are men who don't orgasm or ejaculate due to anxiety, not enough stimulation, erectile dysfunction, or certain meds like antidepressants. Then there is *anejaculation*, which is when a man can orgasm but not ejaculate. This occurs most often in men who've had their prostates removed because of cancer.

RELATED TERMS:
allorgasmia, erotophilic/erotophobic, ithyphallophobia, orgasm, zelophobia

Q: What does **asexuality** actually mean?

A: Ever been crushing on someone who, oddly, did not give off a sexual vibe? Maybe you chalked it up to them simply not being interested or possibly gay? Well, there's another explanation. An asexual person lacks a sex drive, according to Courtney D'Allaird, the coordinator for the Gender and Sexuality Resource Center at the University at Albany. Asexual people may feel attraction, but they don't have the desire to act on it sexually. Unlike celibacy, which is a choice to give up sex, being asexual is an orientation, like being gay or straight, according to the Asexual Visibility and Education Network (AVEN). Asexual people still crave connections with people and often form romantic relationships with others—they have the same emotional needs as any other person, they just don't necessarily want to exchange bodily fluids. Although stats are hard to come by, one study suggests that 1 percent of the population is asexual.

When you're asexual, "you might want to partner with someone forever and be romantic and emotionally intimate, but you don't experience the drive to be physically intimate," explains D'Allaird. The AVEN website notes that asexual people partner with other asexuals as well as with sexual people. Also, the site notes that asexuals can identify as lesbian, gay, bisexual, or straight.

The LGBTQ Center at the University of North Carolina at Chapel Hill states that even though they are frequently aligned, romantic attraction can be different from sexual attraction or asexuality with variations including:

- **aromantic:** individuals who do not experience romantic attraction toward individuals of any gender(s)

- **biromantic:** romantic attraction toward males and females

- **demiromantic:** an individual who does not experience romantic attraction until after a close emotional bond has been formed; people who refer to themselves as demiromantic may choose to further specify the gender(s) of those they are attracted to (e.g., *demi-homoromantic*)

- **demisexual:** those who do not experience primary sexual attraction but may experience secondary sexual attraction after a close emotional connection has already formed

- **gray-A, gray-asexual, gray-sexual:** individuals who feel as though their sexuality falls somewhere on the spectrum of sexuality between asexuality and sexuality

- **gray-romantic:** individuals who do not often experience romantic attraction

- **heteroromantic:** romantic attraction toward persons of a different gender

- **homoromantic:** romantic attraction toward persons of the same gender

- **panromantic:** romantic attraction toward persons of every gender

- **polyromantic:** romantic attraction toward multiple people at once, but not all, genders

RELATED TERMS: *androsexuality, bisexuality, cisgender, gay, gender, genderqueer, heterosexuality/homosexuality, lesbian, nonbinary, pansexuality, transgender, queer*

autofellatio

While few guys out there have the physical dexterity to do this kind of "hot yoga" move, man's quest to blow himself goes way back. In 1948, according to Slate.com, sex researcher Alfred Kinsey noted that while only two or three out of every 1,000 males can do it, a "considerable portion" of young adolescent men attempt autofellatio or self-fellatio. Today it's a popular porn subgenre, with one PornHub "self-suck" video having well over a million views.

RELATED TERMS: *blow job, fellatio, masturbation, oral sex, penis*

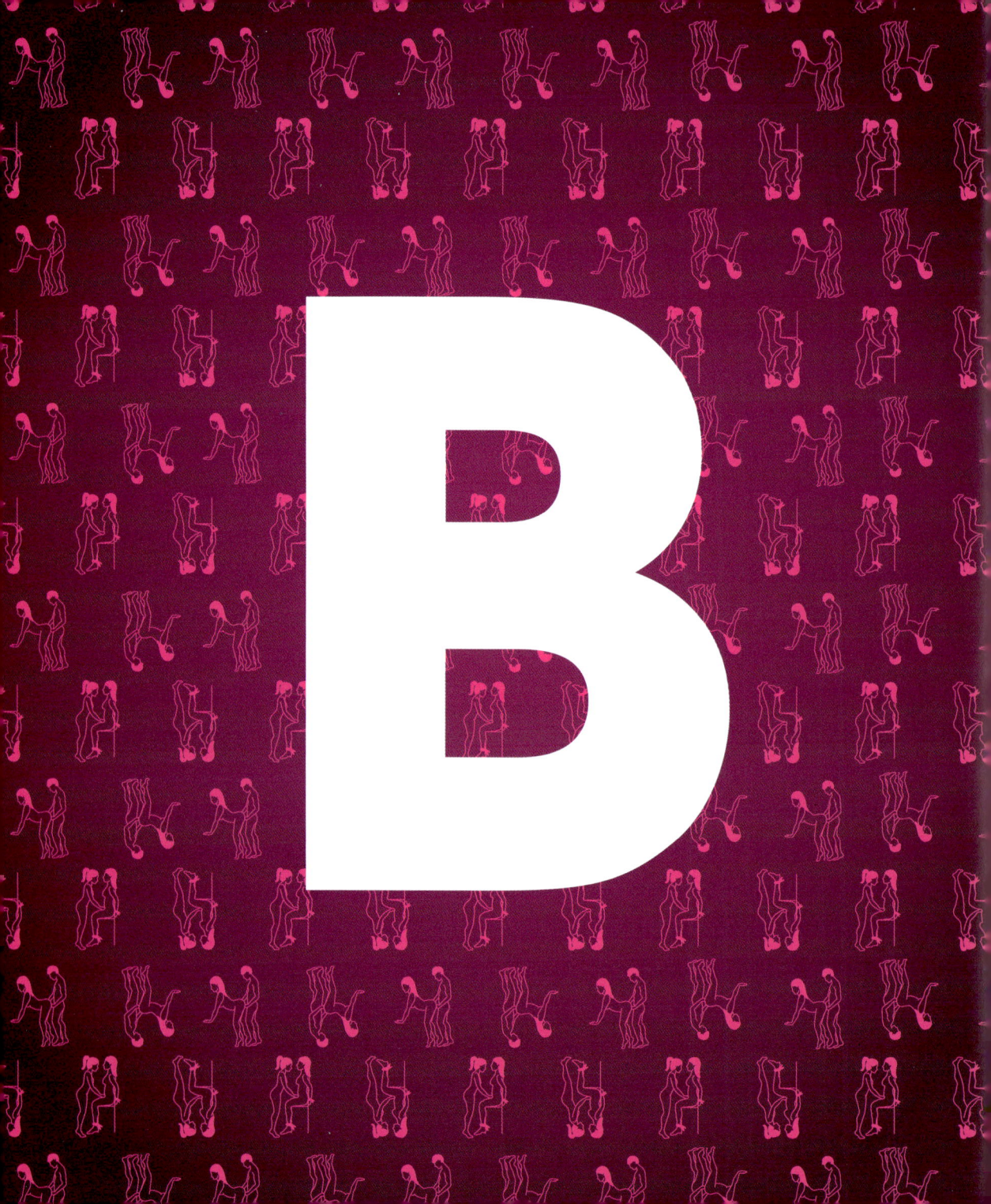

balls

You've got to give testicles their props—the organs that sit in the scrotum under the penis are hardworking little sorry, guys) dudes, making sperm and producing testosterone for the male body. But beyond the basics, here are some fun stuff you might not know about them:

- **Testicles can produce 1,500 sperms cells in one minute** and more than two million in a day.

- **Balls are about seven degrees Fahrenheit cooler** than the rest of the body to ensure that sperm don't overheat.

- *Hum balls* **is the sex move where you put his balls in your mouth** and, you guessed it, hum a little tune. For many guys, the gentle vibration feels well . . . *amazeballs*. (Sorry, we couldn't resist.)

- **Scrotum skin is made from the same type of tissue as the labia majora,** so stroking his sack should give him a feeling similar to what you experience when having your outer labia caressed.

- *Teabagging* **has nothing to do with drinking a nice cuppa** and is all about getting a little bit kinky. Specifically, it's when a man puts his scrotum into the mouth or onto the face of his partner— similar to the act of dipping a tea bag into water. Sex experts like Jessica Drake prefer the term "consensual ball play."

- **Don't worry if your guy's *guys* seem uneven.** One testicle is usually bigger and hangs lower than the other, and for most men, it's the left one, as research published in the journal *Nature* states. Scientists aren't totally sure what determines which ball hangs lower and why the balls don't just hang right next to each other. Some believe it's to keep them from getting too warm, which can harm the sperm inside.

B

TESTICLES CAN PRODUCE 1,500 SPERM CELLS IN ONE MINUTE.

- **Wonder why guys sometimes vomit when they take a hard hit to the balls?** It's because the testes are originally formed in the stomach and even after they descend, there are sensitive nerve pathways still connected, causing a visceral reaction there.

- **Did you know that balls have a built-in bungee cord?** "The *cremaster*, which lines the inside of the scrotum and extends into the groin, controls testicular contractions," explains Barbara Bartlik, MD, a psychiatrist and sex therapist at Weill Cornell Medical College in New York City. "It works kind of like a bungee cord, pulling the testicles upward in response to cold and releasing them when the temperature changes." This magic muscle also responds to sexual stimulation, causing his boys to contract when he's about to orgasm. "The closer a man is to climaxing, the more his testicles recede," explains Debra Fromer, MD, an assistant attending urologist at Hackensack University Medical Center in New Jersey. In turn, pulling down on his balls when you're in the midst of passion delays ejaculation, prolonging his pleasure.

- **Other names for balls include** *bollocks*, *boys*, *cojones*, *dangly bits*, *family jewels*, *gonads* or *nads* (though this can also apply to ovaries), *jingle bells*, *nuts*, and *stones*.

★ RELATED TERMS:
blue balls, genitalia, M-zone, penis, teabagging

bareback

Riding a horse bareback means you're not using a saddle. Riding a person bareback means you're having sex without a condom, which can be risky since it increases chances of STIs and pregnancy. While the term is applicable to couples of any sexual orientation, it's often used in the gay community to describe unprotected anal sex.

RELATED TERMS:
anal, condoms, fuck, sexual intercourse, STI

BDSM

Thanks to *Fifty Shades of Grey*, this abbreviation is pretty common these days. According to Calvert, the BDSM and fetish expert for GameLink, an adult entertainment and e-commerce company, BDSM is an umbrella term that encompasses a wide variety of sexual behaviors and lifestyles and can refer to any or all of the following: bondage and discipline; dominance and submission; sadism and masochism.

The National Coalition for Sexual Freedom (NCSF) describes the practices that often fall within a BDSM lifestyle. Examples include whipping and spanking but also golden showers (the act of one person peeing on another), breath play (any behavior that controls a person's breath, such as choking), and cock-and-ball torture (exactly what it sounds like). BDSM practitioners can experiment with any combination of power-play dynamics. Just because a person enjoys bondage, however, doesn't necessarily mean they enjoy masochism, and vice versa. With BDSM, a person can totally cherry-pick what they like and choose their own adventure. If you're going to give it a test drive, says Calvert. However, just because someone is in a submissive role doesn't mean they don't have control over their own sexual experience. "There's an understanding that it's all a game and that the person who's being submissive has the power to end the game," she adds.

● **Sadism and masochism:** Sadists enjoy giving pain and masochists enjoy receiving it, so pain is incorporated into sexual acts for people who engage in S&M. Pain ranges from very soft, like open-palm slapping, to heavy impact, like using a bullwhip, which can leave marks on the body. (If you're squeamish, stop reading now.) Calvert notes that some of the more extreme forms of S&M play include (yikes!) needle play, electrical play, piercing play, medical play with sutures, and cutting play. Basically, using needles, electric shocks, etc., to stimulate parts of each other's bodies.

✱ **RELATED TERMS:** *consent, kink, masochist, rough sex, safe word*

bisexuality

According to GLAAD, a LGBTQ media advocacy organization, someone who is bisexual "has the capacity to form enduring physical, romantic, and/or emotional attractions to those of the same gender or to those of another gender."

But bisexuality can be challenging, as there are a lot of misconceptions within the LGBTQ community as well as the straight community, according to Courtney D'Allaird, coordinator for the Gender and Sexuality Resource Center at the University at Albany.

Bisexuals sometimes get an unwarranted reputation for promiscuity, says D'Allaird. Also, people often assume that bisexuals are actually just gay and haven't come out yet. But hopefully as people understand more about the fluidity of gender and sexuality, any prejudices or confusion will disappear.

✱ **RELATED TERMS:** *androsexuality, asexuality, cisgender, gay, gender, genderqueer, heterosexuality/ homosexuality, lesbian, nonbinary, pansexuality, transgender, queer*

B

blow job

Oral sex performed on a man—i.e., when you put a guy's penis in your mouth and proceed to suck and lick it—is called a *blow job*, *giving head*, *fellatio*, or *going down* on someone.

Jessica Drake, a sex educator and founder of the *Guide to Wicked Sex*, recommends starting with your hands rather than going right for his penis with your mouth. "Incorporate a lot of different things all at one time. It's not all about sucking the head of his penis. It's more about worshipping the entire area. Run your hands up and down his thighs, pet his penis, do some manipulation with your hand, squeeze it a bit, and feel it as the blood flow starts to get going," she says.

If he hasn't ejaculated after all that "worshipping," you can be creative with your mouth, but "err on the side of caution" with how much suction you apply, says Drake. Switch techniques—and hence, sensations—frequently, so the excitement can build. You can also use dirty talk to elicit feedback. If you're into what you're doing, your partner will be, too.

DRAKE SAYS MEN HAVE TOLD HER THAT THE THREE MOST IMPORTANT THINGS TO TAKE INTO CONSIDERATION WHEN GIVING A BLOW JOB ARE:

- No teeth
- Lots of lubricant from either spit or edible lubricant
- Enthusiasm

Not loving the idea of a penis in your mouth? Definitely feel free to do something else instead.

Also remember that there are still plenty of health risks to giving blow jobs and you can still get STIs. So using a condom is a smart idea.

If you decide to take a blow

job to completion, that age-old question will likely arise in your mind: *Spit or swallow?* There's really no right answer. Drake estimates that about half the men she's encountered couldn't care less if you swallow their semen. "I think that swallowing [is] something that adult movies have definitely made to be the expectation, but I think it's important [for men] to get permission. If men are going to come, they should give their partner a heads-up, so to speak," says Drake. "If you're going to try it, do it all in one gulp and see how that is for you. If you're going to spit, do it discreetly. No one wants to think their bodily fluids are disgusting to a partner."

RELATED TERMS:
cum, deep throating, ejaculation, fellatio, foreplay, orgasm, oral sex, penis, Z-job

yes, **blue balls** are a thing.

Ever heard a guy claim you've given him blue balls? Well, you may have, but don't worry too much about it. The discomfort from a prolonged state of sexual arousal is real for some men, but blue balls won't seriously harm a guy.

When a dude is physically turned on, blood flows to his penis, which is what gives him an erection. Blood also flows to his testicles, causing them to swell. If he doesn't ejaculate, there is a buildup of pressure, and his supersensitive balls feel the brunt of it. But, according to Dr. James Kashanian, MD, a urologist at New York–Presbyterian Hospital Cornell, "there is no risk of irreversible damage."

The sensation can range from a mild ache to worse-than-getting-kicked-in-the-crotch pain. Bottom line: It's not dangerous, and he can deal with the situation, whether that means giving himself a helping hand or just waiting it out. The blood will eventually drain, and any discomfort will disappear on its own.

Dr. Kashanian adds this interesting tidbit: "The color blue seems to have originated from an idea that the scrotum may appear to have a bluish tinge after a prolonged period of sexual arousal, although this has never been substantiated in medical literature. The term could just as easily represent the feeling of the testes feeling bruised, or 'black and blue.'"

RELATED TERMS: *balls, genitalia*

B

10 things you might not know about your **breasts**

1. Bras have been around for a very long time. Ancient Greek women wrapped bandages around their girls to give them the support they needed. The first sports bra was invented in the third century B.C. Today, there are more than four million new bras produced every day, and yet 8 out of 10 women are probably wearing the wrong size.

2. In one study, 50 percent of mothers found breastfeeding erotic. A lot of them felt guilty about it, but it's totally normal. Hormones released during nursing might turn you on.

3. There are four different types of nipples. They are *normal* (where the nipples stick out a bit from the areola), *flat* (where the nipple blends into the areola but can extend when aroused), *puffy* (where the areola is raised up off the breast), or *inverted* (where the nipples fold into the areola). Just as skin tones can vary from person to person, so can the color of nipples and areolae.

4. Your breasts are more prone to dry skin than any other body part. Because your breasts stretched when you hit puberty, they have thinner skin than the rest of your body, making them more likely to become dry than other places. And yes, even your nipples need a moisturizer.

5. Six percent of people have an extra nipple. Called a *supernumerary nipple*, some evidence suggests that they more commonly occur on the left side of the body.

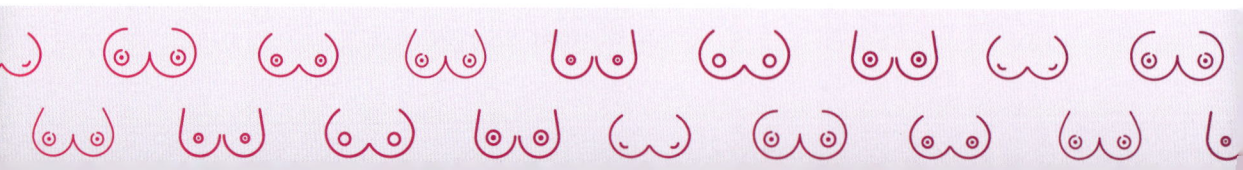

6. It's not just men who're fascinated by your rack.
Other women stare at your breasts a lot. A study using eye-tracking devices showed that while guys spent more time staring at your breasts, women also spent plenty of time watching your breasts and not your face. So, everyone—eyes up.

7. Don't expect one breast to be exactly the same as the other.
For two-thirds of women, the pair doesn't match—many have a larger left breast. But if your seemingly identical twins suddenly become fraternal, head to your doctor. You could have an infection or worse.

8. Your breast size changes all the time.
You can go up as much as a full cup size (holy shit!) at certain points in your period cycle, which can be a good thing or a bad thing depending on whether or not you love wearing button-down shirts.

9. Breasts can weigh up to 20 pounds or more.
This gives new understanding to why they're sometimes called "melons."

10. Sleeping facedown can change the shape of your breasts over time.
The best snooze style for your girls? On your side, with a pillow providing support as you doze.

★ **RELATED TERMS:** *boobgasm, nipples*

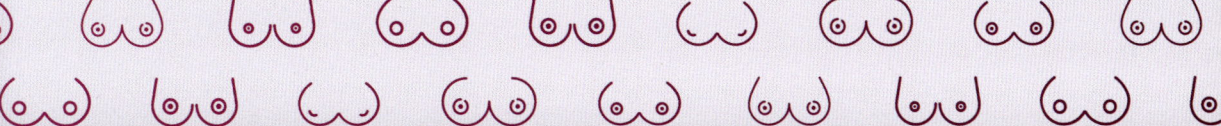

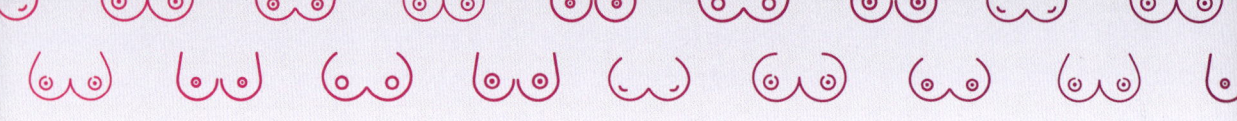

101 DIFFERENT NAMES FOR boo

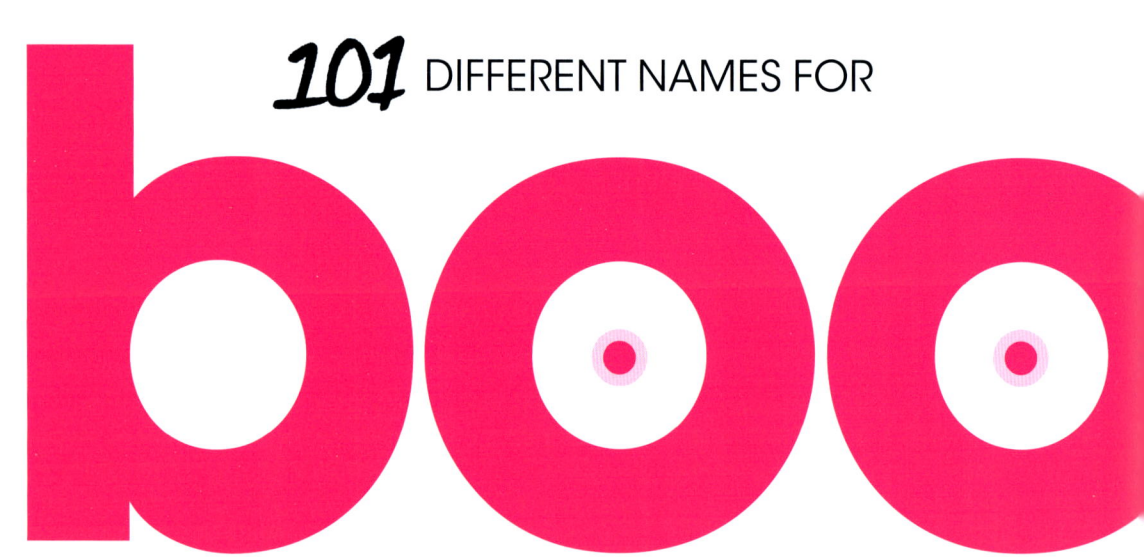

Boobs, the twins, titties, breasts—we all probably have quite a few names we like to use when referring to our baps, and now D–K-cup lingerie expert Curvy Kate has finally put them all in one hilarious list.

1. Breasts
2. Boobs
3. Mammary Glands
4. Boobies
5. Tits

SOME FOOD-RELATED NAMES

6. Fiery Biscuits (really!?)
7. Melons
8. Baps
9. Coconuts
10. Yorkshire Puddings
11. Bangers
12. Cream Pies
13. Iced Gems
14. Bacon Hangers (we can't even)
15. Chips and Dips
16. Fried Eggs
17. Cantaloupes

MILKY VIBES

18. "She drank her school milk"
19. Milk Monsters
20. Milkers

RANDOM CELEBRITY NAMES

21. Brad Pitts
22. Danny DeVitos

DOUBLE ACTS

23. The Twins
24. Minnie and Mickey
25. Phil and Lil
26. Mary-Kate and Ashley
35. Udders
36. Spaniel's Ears
37. Mosquito Bites

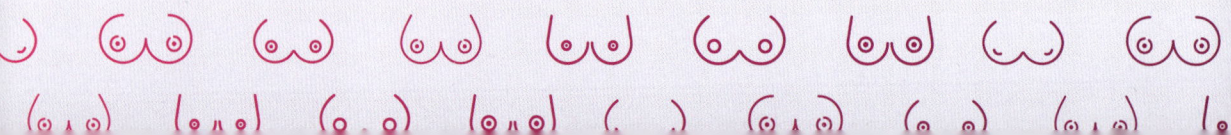

bs!

CUTE NAMES

38. Noogies
39. Babs
40. Lills
41. The Girls
42. Buds
43. Bips

PRETTY MUCH EVERYTHING ELSE

44. Norks
45. Chebs
46. Maracas
47. Slammers
48. Tig Ol' Bitties
49. Chebblies
50. Wabs
51. Funbags
52. Chesticles
53. Jugs
54. Waps
55. Tatas
56. Bazoombas
57. Breasticles
58. Bazookas
59. Mammeries
60. Bristol Cities
61. Cha-Chas
62. Bosoms
63. Jubblies
64. Charlies
65. Juganauts
66. Peaks
67. Knockers
68. Rack
69. Shelf
70. Dongles
71. Nunga Nungas
72. Wangers
73. Swingers
74. Airbags
75. Tatty Bo Jangles
76. Honker Honkers
77. Cans
78. Babylons
79. Bubbalas
80. Nipple Holsters
81. Life Savers
82. Buoyancy Aids
83. Orbs
84. Bongos
85. Watties
86. Bouncers
87. Wagons
88. Globes
89. Shoulder Boulders
90. Hooters
91. Muchachas

GRIM NAMES

92. Titties
93. Man Boobs
94. Fleshy Mounds
95. Upper Bollocks
96. TBs (Top Bollocks)
97. Dirty Pillows
98. Naughty Pillows
99. Two Old Socks
100. Aspirin on an Ironing Board
101. Mud Flaps

Q: Can i really have a boobgasm?

A: The answer may be... *YASS*. A study from the *Journal of Sexual Medicine* found that a little nipple play before and during sex can enhance arousal. The effect? The potential for a more intense climax. More shocking: Some women have even reported having orgasms from breast play alone... lucky ladies!

What's behind those boobgasms? Mostly your brain, says Barry Komisaruk, PhD, a neuroscientist at Rutgers University. "Nipple stimulation activates the same part of the sensory cortex as clitoral and vaginal stimulation do," he says. Or, in plain-speak: Rubbing your headlights ignites your noggin's feel-good center. And when your upper and lower parts are engaged simultaneously, it can lead to a mind-blowing release.

There's no wrong turn on the road toward nipple euphoria. Just remember to communicate and practice with your partner to figure out what makes you happy, says Jill McDevitt, PhD, a resident sexologist at lubricant company Swiss Navy. Start by having your partner slowly trace their fingers around your areolae, inching ever closer to the center. If your nips get hard or feel tingly, the moves are working. "Have your mate cup your breasts and use their fingers to gently squeeze your nipples," says McDevitt. Or tell them to lap your nips with a little tongue before gently kissing and sucking them.

Some advanced experimentation can prompt an even more explosive boobgasm. Try circling your nips with a small vibrator, a warming lubricant, ice cubes, or—for an extreme adventure—nipple clamps. That said, don't force it. If your girls are sore, tender, or aching for any reason, stimulating them is more likely to prompt an ouch than an O. Respect your twins by letting them act as passive bystanders until they're ready to join the party again.

RELATED TERMS:
breasts, nipple clamps, nipples, orgasm

butt plug

An anal sex toy shaped like a teardrop, it's meant to be placed, or "plugged," into your butthole. The base of a butt plug is designed to be wide so it doesn't get sucked into and "lost" in your rectum, because that would be, well, a bummer.

According to Tristan Taormino, a sex educator and author of *The Ultimate Guide to Anal Sex for Women*, "[A butt plug] is designed to go in your ass and stay there. If you like in-and-out penetration, then you want a dildo." (It's also worth trying a strap-on, which is a dildo with a harness that you wear around your waist.) She says that people experience pleasure differently—some like a feeling of fullness, which is what a butt plug accomplishes. When inserting a butt plug into yourself or your partner, use lubrication, always go slow, and ask questions to see if the sensation is doing it for them.

Taormino also explains that some of the nerve endings in the rectum respond to pressure rather than massage. Butt plugs can be used as a "warm-up" for other sorts of anal play, like using dildos, larger toys, and anal intercourse, or they can be left in while you perform other sex acts. If interested in anal play, start out with a smaller plug and work your way up.

RELATED TERMS: *anal, anal play, double penetration, lube, pegging, sex toys*

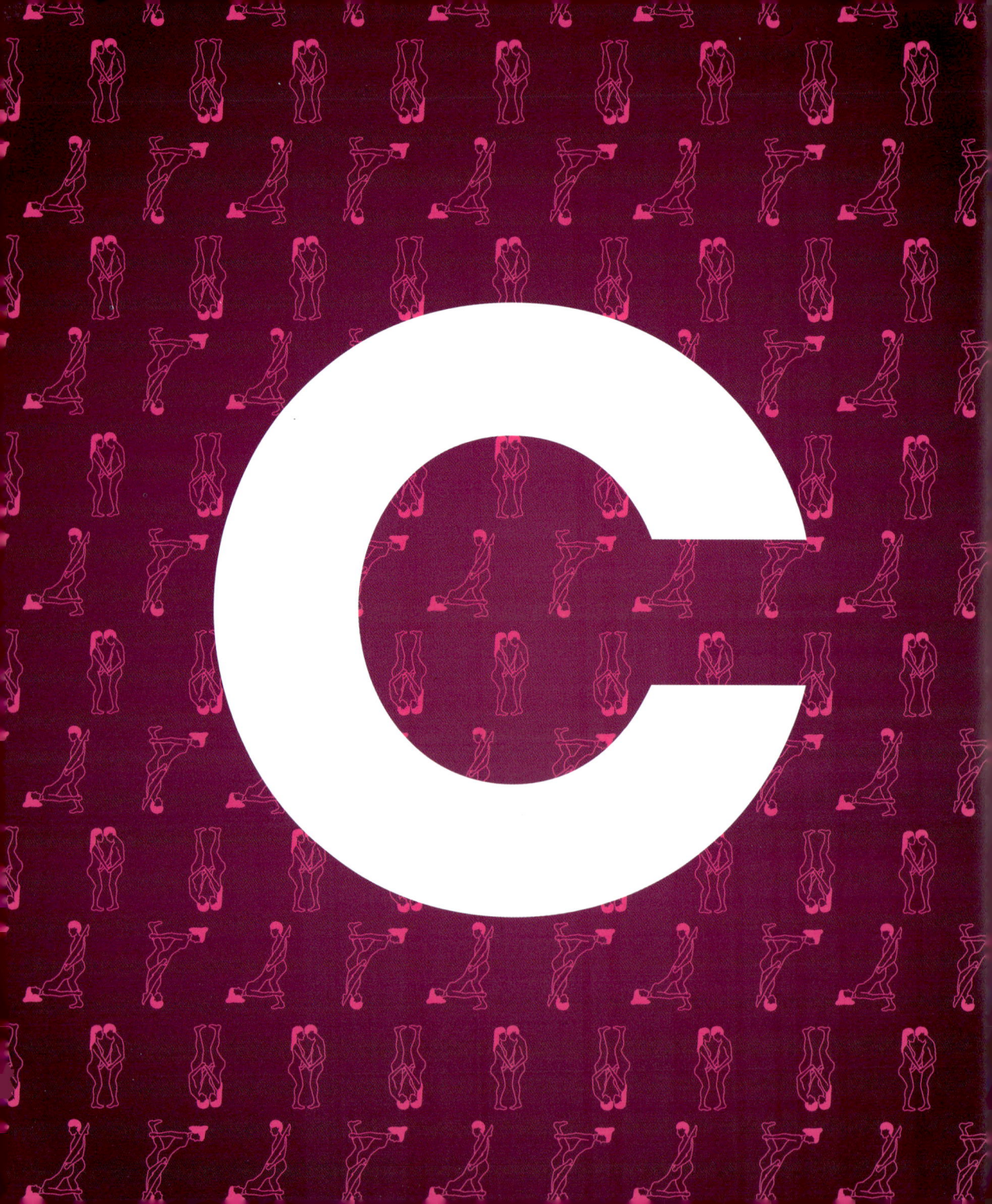

circumcision

Every penis is its own unique snowflake. They can be big, small, thin, fat, cute, and quirky. They can also be circumcised (cut) or have full-on foreskin (uncut). Here's what you need to know!

Circumcision—the removal of the foreskin of the penis to reveal the head—usually happens when a boy is a baby, though some brave men opt for it in adulthood. It's popular in the US, with 77 percent of male babies born in hospitals being circumcised, according to a review by the Mayo Clinic. It's also practiced in Judaism and Islam as a religious ritual.

Even though the majority of male babies are circumcised, the rate of newborn circumcision in the US has declined by 10 percent since 1979. This is due, in part, to an increasing amount of activism around the topic that has made parents question whether the procedure is necessary or disfiguring.

• But is it healthier?
According to the World Health Organization (WHO), one of the benefits of circumcision is a lower risk of HIV transmission. WHO states, "There is compelling evidence that male circumcision reduces the risk of heterosexually acquired HIV infection in men by approximately 60 percent."

• Can it affect a man's sexual pleasure?
James Kashanian, MD, a urologist at New York–Presbyterian Hospital Cornell, says he's had men report both an increase and a decrease in sensation during sex after circumcision. So even though some uncut men swear that sex is better for them because their equipment is all natural, that hasn't been proven. And to make this all about women's pleasure for a second: There's no difference in sensation for the woman.

• Does it make for a cleaner penis?
The gunk that can accumulate under a man's foreskin is called *smegma*, and it's an oft-cited reason that proponents of circumcision use to support the practice. But with proper cleaning and hygiene, it's not an issue.

• Can a circumcision be reversed?
No, says Dr. Kashanian, but a skin graft can be added in situations where a circumcision is botched and too much skin is removed.

• How is a circumcision done?
Obviously this is not something you should try at home. But for the morbidly curious, a circumcision is performed by first applying a topical anesthesia to the penis. Once the penis is numb, the foreskin is opened and separated from the glans and then cut off.

✱ **RELATED TERMS:**
penis, STIs, uncircumcised

C

CIS IS NOT A "FAKE" WORD AND IS NOT A SLUR.

cisgender

The University of Nebraska Omaha Gender and Sexuality Resource Center defines cisgender as "an adjective that means 'identifies as their sex assigned at birth,' derived from the Latin word meaning 'on the same side.'"

THE CENTER ALSO NOTES THAT:

- *Cisgender* does not indicate biology, gender expression, or sexuality/sexual orientation.

- A cisgender/cis person is not transgender.

- In discussions regarding trans issues, one would differentiate between women who are trans and women who aren't by saying *trans women* and *cis women*.

- *Cis* is not a "fake" word and is not a slur.

✻ RELATED TERMS:
androsexuality, asexuality, bisexuality, gay, gender, genderqueer, heterosexuality/ homosexuality, lesbian, nonbinary, pansexuality, transgender, queer

4 things to know about your clitoris

Your clit is badass! It's the magical carpet ride to almost all your orgasms.

Considering all it does, do you really know enough about it? Don't worry, we've got you covered. Dr. Emily Nagoski, director of wellness education at Smith College and author of *Come as You Are: The Surprising New Science That Will Transform Your Sex Life*, shares key things about your favorite body part ever.

The clitoris isn't just the nub at the top of your vulva. Even though it looks like it begins and ends there, the clitoris actually extends all the way down to the entrance of the vagina, and has internal structures as well.

Those same internal clitoral structures might actually be what we think of as the G-spot. In sonograms, researchers looked at how the inside of our bodies change during sex. They found that during penetration, the vagina flexes in a way that makes the penis rub through the vaginal wall and onto the internal structures of the clitoris, which people often think is G-spot stimulation. It can vary from woman to woman, but for some, when they experience G-spot orgasms, it's actually just an internal extension of the clit.

Not all clit stimulation feels good. We're all told that the clit is the only organ designed purely for pleasure, but that's not true. It's actually designed for sensation. And if you're not turned on, any kind of clitoral stimulation might not feel good. Basically, it's not a magic doorbell that you can press any time of day and have everything open up perfectly. You have to be in the mood first for magic to happen.

Clitoris size varies. In the web series *If Our Bodies Could Talk*, host James Hamblin notes that the dimensions of a clit can range from 0.09 inches (0.23 cm) to 0.17 inches (0.43 cm) wide to 0.15 inches (0.38 cm) to 0.26 inches (0.66 cm) long.

NOTE: A large clit isn't necessarily more or less sensitive than a small one.

✱ RELATED TERMS:
G-spot, genitalia, labia, vagina, vulva

ms

Whether you love 'em or hate 'em, using condoms continues to be one of the key ways to avoid STI's and unwanted pregnancy. But how much do you really know about them?

Goodyear's rubber vulcanization process led to the first rubber condom being produced in 1855, which is why present-day latex condoms are sometimes called "rubbers" by people like your dad and grandfather.

◉ **Condoms really haven't been redesigned since they were invented.** Latex condoms were introduced around the 1920s and, despite advances made with bumps and ridges, have remained largely unchanged.

◉ **Condoms (on average) don't really affect the quality of sex.** Surveys show that couples were just as satisfied with sex whether or not they were using condoms. So considering that condoms are 98 percent effective at preventing pregnancy and make sex a hell of a lot safer, "it doesn't feel good" isn't an excuse not to use one.

◉ **Your parents are less likely to use condoms than you are.** Sorry to put that image in your mind, but couples over 40 are the least likely to use condoms for a variety of reasons, including they often are less worried about getting pregnant and are having sex with a committed partner.

◉ **Condom use may change with your relationship status.** On average, 25 percent of couples use condoms, while 33 percent of single people use them.

◉ **Women account for almost half of condom sales.** Even though they go on penises, women account for at least 40 percent of condom purchases. Which is good, because you should pretty much always have them on hand.

✱ **RELATED TERMS:**
bareback, consent, fuck, sexual intercourse, STI, yes means yes

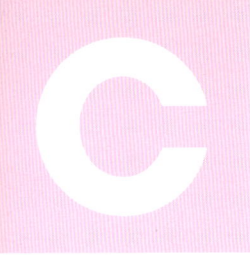

consensual nonmonogamy

Relationships that are "consensually nonmonogamous (CNM)" are ones in which, according to Dr. Justin Lehmiller, "the partners involved agree that having more than one sexual and/or romantic partner at the same time is permissible."

There are many variations and terms associated with CNM relationships, but here are a few you should know:

- **anchor partner:**
the person you've probably been with the longest and may live with

- **open relationship:**
a committed relationship between two partners who also sleep with other people (but may have to get permission in advance)

- **polyamory:**
the practice of maintaining romantic relationships with multiple committed partners

- **polycule:**
an extended family comprised of polyamorous relationships (e.g., your boyfriend's girlfriends may be in your polycule)

- **relationship escalator:**
the arc of a traditional relationship from cohabitation to marriage and kids; aka a ride many poly people are trying to get off

- **solo poly:**
when you have more than one partner but no "main" partner

- **throuple:**
like a couple but with three people

- **unicorn:**
a bisexual woman who has sex with heterosexual married couples

★ **RELATED TERMS:**
polyamory, monogamy

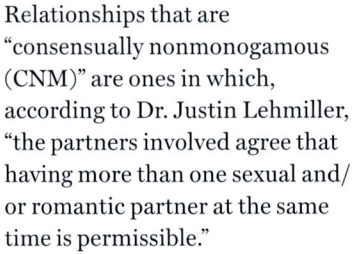

> CONSENT IS AN AGREEMENT BETWEEN PARTICIPANTS TO ENGAGE IN SEXUAL ACTIVITY.

consent

We all know that "yes means yes." But that doesn't mean there aren't questions about how consent works in daily life. According to RAINN (Rape, Abuse & Incest National Network), "Consent is an agreement between participants to engage in sexual activity. Consent does not have to be verbal, but verbally agreeing to different sexual activities can help both you and your partner respect each other's boundaries. ... When you're engaging in sexual activity, consent is about communication. And it should happen every time. Giving consent for one activity, one time, does not mean giving consent for increased or recurring sexual contact. For example, agreeing to kiss someone doesn't give that person permission to remove your clothes. Having sex with someone in the past doesn't give that person permission to have sex with you again in the future."

RAINN DESCRIBES OTHER COMMON POINTS ABOUT CONSENT:

○ **"You can change your mind at any time.**
You can withdraw consent at any point if you feel uncomfortable. It's important to clearly communicate to your partner that you are no longer comfortable with this activity and wish to stop. The best way to ensure both parties are comfortable with any sexual activity is to talk about it.

○ **"Positive consent can look like this:**
→ Communicating when you change the type or degree of sexual activity with phrases like, 'Is this okay?'
→ Explicitly agreeing to certain activities, either by saying 'yes' or another affirmative statement, like 'I'm open to trying.'
→ Using physical cues to let the other person know you're comfortable with taking things to the next level.

○ **"Consent does NOT look like this:**
→ Refusing to acknowledge 'no.'
→ Assuming that wearing certain clothes, flirting, or kissing are invitations for anything more.
→ Someone being under the legal age of consent, as defined by the state.
→ Someone being incapacitated because of drugs or alcohol.
→ Pressuring someone into sexual activity by using fear or intimidation.
→ Assuming you have permission to engage in a sexual act because you've done it in the past."

yes, **consent** can make sex sexier

With all the recent ideas around how to properly demonstrate consent, it can start to feel like another insurmountable chore that makes sex way less fun, explains Emily Morse, sexologist and host of the podcast *Sex with Emily*. The truth is, she says, "Consent done right will actually enhance your sex life on many levels."

"Foreplay," says Morse, "is a crucial part of gauging sexual satisfaction, especially for women. Incorporating consent into your 'sex talk' by describing in detail what you'd like to happen later, next, or in the moment can be the hottest and most efficient way to make sure you're getting what you desire, and it keeps you from engaging in any unwanted activities or regrets. For example, saying something like, 'I love when you kiss my neck and ask me what I want you to do to me,' can be really hot and signals to your partner that asking before doing is actually a turn-on. Then it becomes a sexy back-and-forth, where both of you are completely transparent in what is okay and not okay moving forward. So your ongoing consent is really masked as dirty talk, but with a purpose."

Morse says that talking about sex can be awkward, even for long-time couples. However, conversations about sex can make you more comfortable with your partner during the deed. "Trust is sexy. The more you trust your partner—and the more they trust you—the easier it will be to open up about what feels good, your personal desires and fantasies, and what you *really* want," says Morse.

That said, you do not have to walk on eggshells. According to Morse, "a lot of men and women view consent as an ongoing 'are you okay, is this okay' play-by-play,

> TRUST IS SEXY. THE MORE YOU TRUST YOUR PARTNER— AND THE MORE THEY TRUST YOU— THE EASIER IT WILL BE TO OPEN UP ABOUT WHAT FEELS GOOD, YOUR PERSONAL DESIRES AND FANTASIES, AND WHAT YOU *REALLY* WANT.

when really it's just an exchange of what you both want sexually in the moment—which is really hot. Sure, you're checking in along the way, but if you're using a sexy tone, you'll not only be really turned on but also very present, so it'll be easier to stop something that doesn't feel right in the moment. This also makes it easier to try new things with your partner, because you've already opened up that fun and sexy dialogue."

✳ RELATED TERMS:
dirty talk, foreplay, fuck, safe word, sexual intercourse, yes means yes

C

coregasm

5 PERCENT OF WOMEN EXPERIENCE EXERCISE-INDUCED Os

You've probably heard a story at some point about a friend's cousin's sister-in-law who once had an orgasm while she worked out. And odds are, you laughed it off. But it turns out the exercise-induced O is no urban myth.

A study from Indiana University's Center for Sexual Health Promotion found that this phenomena is legit—and certain exercises are more likely than others to set women off. Researchers discovered that exercises that target your core—planks, crunches, etc.—are more likely to give women what they termed *coregasms*.

A previous study found that at least 5 percent of women experience exercise-induced Os, and researchers at Indiana University wanted to dig a little deeper. Of the women they surveyed, 40 percent said they'd had at least eleven coregasms in their lives, and the majority of them said they weren't thinking about sex when they happened.

So what caused them?
Forty-five percent of the women said they went over the edge thanks to abdominal exercises, while 19 percent said spinning did it for them. Running and lifting weights also gave some women coregasms. But the ab exercise where you support your arms in padded arm rests and lift your knees toward your chest caused the most Os.

✳ **RELATED TERM:**
orgasm

Q: What is **cosplay?**

A: Short for *costume play*, cosplay is different from, say, dressing up like a sexy cat on Halloween. According to Ela Darling, a cosplay aficionado, cosplay simply means dressing up as your favorite character from a comic book, movie, or novel, and taking on the persona of that character.

As events like Comic-Con have exploded in popularity, so has the phenomenon of adults dressing like wizards in public. Cosplay can be sexual or nonsexual, depending on the context. Dressing as Wonder Woman and doing a striptease for your boyfriend? Sexual. Dressing as Gandalf for a *Lord of the Rings* viewing party? Whatever the opposite of sexy is.

Darling explains that at its core, cosplay is simply "a way to celebrate your fandom." So it's not necessarily a sexual thing. Consider the context and surroundings before assuming a costume is an invitation for sexual attention. A lot of fangirls who participate in cosplay feel like they are oversexualized. Darling notes that at events like Comic-Con, women who dress up "hate being mistaken for any kind of adult entertainer. They're already in a place surrounded mostly by men who are not always great at keeping boundaries."

FURRIES

You can't really talk about cosplay without mentioning furries, a subculture of people who like to dress up in animal costumes, often as a sexual fetish. Like cosplay, the furry trend came out of nerd culture. As with almost every fandom, there is a pornographic side, in this case known as *yiff*. There are furry dating sites and furry conventions and, yes, even furry sex scandals. At the heart of the furry fetish is a sexual desire to dress like an animal character and have sexual relations with other people who do the same.

RELATED TERMS: *fetish, kink*

creampie

When most people think of a creampie, the classic American sweet treat usually comes to mind. But there is another meaning that is way less family-friendly. The nondessert definition of a creampie is when semen visibly drips out of a vagina or anus after a man ejaculates inside a partner during sex.

RELATED TERMS: *anal, ejaculation, semen*

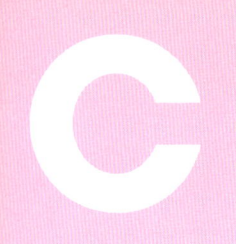

cum

According to Urban Dictionary, it's sticky goo that squirts out of a guy's penis when he becomes sexually aroused." For a more official explanation, see our definition of *semen* on page 173.

RELATED TERMS: *cum shot, ejaculation, facial, jerking off, masturbation, orgasm, pearl necklace, semen*

---

cum shot

Unless you're a budding pornographer or particularly bold when it comes to making sexy videos with your current bae, you probably won't need to stage one of these graphic shots of your own.

Cum shot is a term used in porn that refers to the filmed moment when a man ejaculates, usually on his partner, where the semen can be easily seen. It's also called the *money shot* or *pop shot*. According to Kelly Madison, a *facial*—where a man ejaculates on a woman's face—is the most popular type of cum shot in porn. She notes that in mainstream porn, showing the cum shot is necessary for a shoot to be considered successful. Ugh.

RELATED TERMS:
ejaculation, facial, money shot, orgasm, pearl necklace, semen

cunnilingus

Cunnilingus is a fancy term that means oral sex performed on a woman, though most people don't use it in casual conversation because it has more of a sterile, academic feel. You wouldn't turn to your homegirl at brunch and be like, "My boyfriend gave me excellent cunnilingus last night. Mimosas for everyone!"

Generally the way it works is that the giver uses their lips and tongue to lick, suck, and nibble on a woman's vulva and clitoris. It feels pretty fabulous. Cunnilingus can also be called a bunch of other, more casual slang terms: *eating pussy*, *rug munching*, and *muff diving* are just a few of the more popular (and ridiculous) ones. The point is, it doesn't matter what you call it, as long as you're gettin' it.

According to Lily Cade, a lesbian porn performer who has lots of experience both giving and receiving cunnilingus in her real life and as an actor in girl-on-girl porn, says, "Most girls either want you to suck on [the clitoris], move your tongue in a circle, or move the tongue up and down and sideways." She recommends starting slowly and with a light touch, then working up to more speed and pressure as you get feedback.

RELATED TERMS: *oral sex, orgasm*

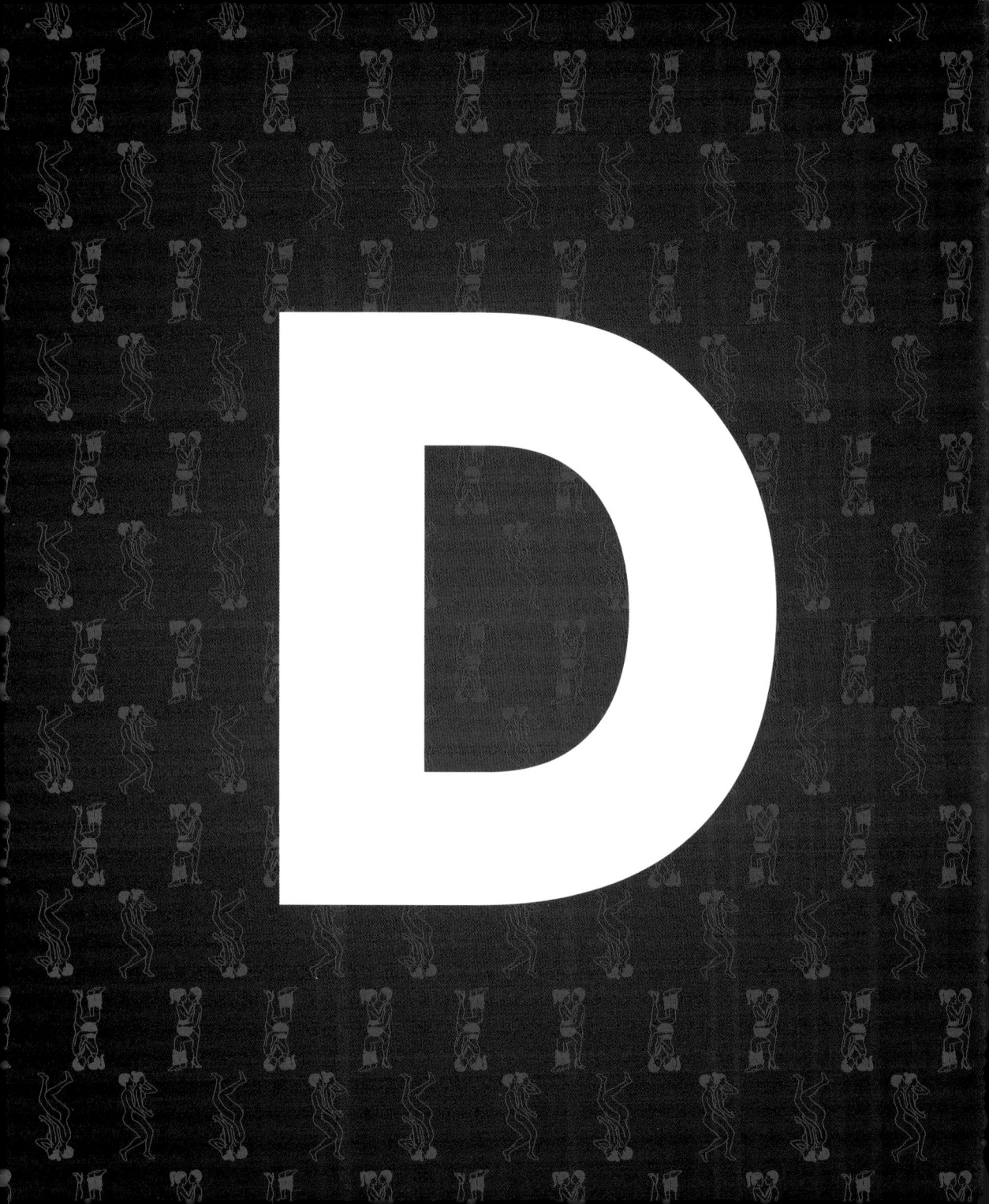

Q: What is **deep-throating?**

A: A term used to describe a type of next-level/more intense blow job.

The way it works is that during the act, the blower puts as much of the penis as they can in their mouth—which is sometimes the whole thing. The penis gets pushed deep into the throat (ergo the name), which can sometimes cause gagging or even vomiting. (Not fun!) Like many popular moves you see in porn, this technique generally feels great for the guy receiving the deep throating but can be super uncomfortable for the person giving head.

Jessica Drake, educator and founder of the *Guide to Wicked Sex*, a series of erotic educational films, says this is definitely an instance to slow your roll and proceed with caution.

"If you're gagging when you're brushing your teeth and tongue, you are not a great candidate," she warns. "It actually requires work and practice, and—contrary to what you see in adult movies—it isn't that easy. There's a large object threatening to cut off your air supply."

When a penis hits the back of your throat, your body's first instinct is to get it out, which is what triggers the gag reflex. However, that also makes you produce a lot of saliva, which will make the whole process easier, as it acts as a natural lubricant.

If you want to feel comfortable with the experience, Drake recommends putting yourself in a position of power so you can control the depth of penetration. It is also important to discuss consent, safe words, and safe signals ahead of time to make sure your partner will withdraw the moment you want him to.

Once the penis is inside your mouth, try to relax your throat muscles as much as possible. To help stay calm and relaxed, remember that you are in control and can stop at any time. Also, the slower you go, the easier it will be.

What if your partner is well-endowed? Wrap your hand around the base of the penis so it can only go so far, Drake advises. Also, if your man is uncircumcised, don't pull the foreskin too far back or it can hurt, as the head of the penis for uncircumcised men can be much more sensitive.

RELATED TERMS:
blow job, circumcision, consent, fellatio, oral sex, safe word

D

Cosmo's Ultimate dicktionary

While you won't come across these terms in your standard college dictionary, here's a cheat sheet full of fun words for various shaft-related situations.

- **Dickstracted** (adj) *dik-strak-ted* / the state of being unable to concentrate after seeing the outline of a guy's impressive manhood through his pants

- **Dicknapped** (v) *dik-napt* / when you have plans with your crew, but your boy entices you to stay in for some hot fun, so you never make it out the door

- **Dickcited** (adj) *dik-si-ted* / the feeling of being amped up to get some action, as in, "I'm seeing Jake tonight. I'm so dickcited!"

- **Dickcicle** (n) *dik-si-kel* / a guy with such a cold heart, he smashes and dashes without so much as a drip of remorse

- **Dickter scale** (n) *dik-ter skal* / a numerical rating for how magical a penis is (e.g., "he's a solid eight"); the phallic equivalent of the Richter scale

- **Dickcision** (n) *dik-si-zhn* / when a dude acts by thinking solely with his D rather than with his actual brain

- **Dick magnet** (n) *dik mag-net* / a woman who attracts any guy she wants without having to say a damn word; the female version of a chick magnet

- **Dickcipline** (n) *dik-s-pln* / when you exercise the willpower not to hook up with a bro, even if you really, really want to

- **Dick flick** (n) *dik flik* / a testosterone-infused blockbuster; typically involves nonstop car chases, over-the-top explosions, and random shots of half-naked women

dildo

This penis-shaped sex toy is designed for penetration to either stay inside the vagina and/or anus or be pushed in and out. Not to be confused with vibrators, as most dildos don't need batteries and won't wiggle and jiggle on their own.

According to the sex-toy retailer Babeland, "Dildo shopping involves a lot of personal preference. Shape, size, texture, style, and color are all up to you.... Materials are one of the most important considerations in choosing a dildo. Nonporous materials like silicone, Pyrex, and stainless steel are the easiest to care for and last much longer than porous materials like jelly rubber or cyberskin."

Some dildo variations include *realistic*, *nonrealistic* (think dolphin/cute bunny rabbit), *double-ended*, and *G-spot stimulating*.

✺ **RELATED TERMS:** *anal play, double penetration, lesbian sex, masturbation, orgasm, pegging, sex toys*

SEX-TOY CARE 101

Keeping your toys clean between playtimes is super important. It's best to read the cleaning directions that came with the toy, since there are different recommendations depending on the materials—but most can be cleaned by washing with soap and warm water. If it's made of glass, Pyrex, stainless steel, or pure silicone, stick it in boiling water for a few minutes (if it doesn't contain a motor, that is).

Remember, though, that porous materials can never be 100 percent sanitized—still wash them, of course, but also put condoms over them if you're using them with multiple partners or if you and your partner aren't having safe, protected sex in the first place.

D dirty

While there's nothing literally messy or unclean about it, dialogue of an overt sexual nature has earned this moniker. For many, it's an effective way to express their desires and introduce new things they want to try. Plus, according to a recent study in the *Journal of Social and Personal Relationships*, people who show signs of sexual communication apprehension enjoy sex less. One way to enjoy sex more? Get comfortable talking—or texting—with your partner about what you want.

That might not come naturally for everyone. In fact, it can feel totally awkward if you're not accustomed to throwing around crass words for bodyparts or vocalizing the specifics of what you want in bed. Even so, it's a skill you might be able to learn, says Tina Horn, an expert on sexy talk who teaches workshops on the topic, and the author of *Sexting: The Grownup's Little Book of Sex Tips for Getting Dirty Digitally*.

DILF

In appreciation of hot-AF dads everywhere, DILF stands for "dad I'd like to fuck." You may have your own list, but popular celeb DILFs include David Beckham, Idris Elba, Tom Hardy, John Legend, Channing Tatum, Justin Timberlake, and Usher.

talk

The first question people usually ask at her dirty talk workshops is, "How do I do it without sounding silly?" According to Horn, the best thing you can say to someone to kick off racy dialogue is "I want you" or "I love it when you . . ." Partners like to know they and their efforts are appreciated. She also provides a list of words to get comfortable using in bed, which include but aren't limited to *come, fuck, bang, suck, hard, wet, yes, no, now,* *slower* and *faster*, *dick*, *clit*, *mouth*, and *ass*. You get the idea. Put them together and see what sexy combos you can come up with.

Another strategy popularized by sex advice expert Dan Savage: Describe to your partner what you're going to do to them, what you are doing to them, and what you just did to them. For example, "Baby, I'm going to climb on top of you and ride you so hard;" "I'm riding you so fucking hard;" "I just rode you so hard."

The dirty talk guidelines used IRL also generally apply to sexting. "When it comes to texting on your phone, G-chatting, or emailing, you have to be very deliberate and very methodical, and really pace yourself," Horn recommends. You can't read any nonverbal cues over a text, so choose your words or emojis carefully.

❋ **RELATED TERMS:**
foreplay, fuck, sexting, sexual intercourse

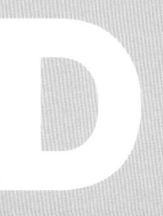

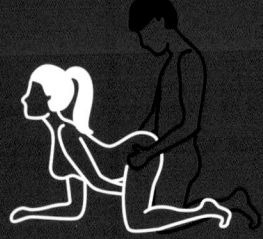

doggy style

Inspired by our furry friends, doggy-style sex involves the receiver on hands and knees, while their partner enters through the vagina or butt from behind with a penis or strap-on . . . you get the idea.

According to sex expert Casey Calvert, "It's one of the most common positions people do, not just in porn but in their own bedrooms, too." Some women find that penetration seems deeper in this position, which could be a plus or minus depending on what you like.

The basic version involves getting comfortable on your hands and knees and having your partner enter you from behind while on his knees (and communicate if it's too hard/too soft/too anything).

MAKE IT HOTTER:

◉ Find something to hold onto, like a headboard, so you get some leverage and can control the force of his thrusting.

◉ Grab a vibrator or use your hand to give your clitoris some attention while your partner is busy thrusting. Or put a pillow under your pelvis and rub your way to clitoral bliss.

◉ Try having the receiving partner stand and bend over a chair or table while their partner—also standing—enters from behind.

◉ You can also play with the angle of your booty to see how it affects penetration and sensation. Try arching your back, sticking your butt up higher, or lying completely flat on your stomach.

RELATED TERMS: *fuck, positions, sexual intercourse*

double penetration

Ever considered trying to double your pleasure by taking a penis in the front and back doors at the same time? Traditionally, you need two penises and their accompanying men to anally and vaginally penetrate you simultaneously—but you can also swap that second dude for a dildo. Or even go guy-free and try a double-headed dildo by yourself.

Here, sexologist and sex educator Dr. Sayaka Adachi shares her tips on how to approach double penetration, which, let's face it, can be pretty intimidating. "One can try first with toys to see if that's something you like. Start out with a butt plug while being vaginally penetrated [by a partner]. It's good to practice having two things inside you before moving into having two guys." According to Dr. Sayaka, some people prefer to put the bigger object in the vagina and smaller one in the anus—it's your call.

✸ **RELATED TERMS:** *anal, anal play, lube, sex toys*

dry orgasm

More formally known as *retrograde ejaculation*, this term describes when a man's semen goes back toward the bladder rather than out the penis during climax—potentially rendering him infertile. According to the Mayo Clinic Patient Care and Health Info website, retrograde ejaculation can be caused by many things, including certain types of medication, surgery, or nerve damage. If your dude is dry orgasming, he should get himself checked out.

✸ **RELATED TERMS:** *ejaculation, orgasm, penis, semen*

> **DTF**
> An acronym for "down to fuck" that you'll see on dating apps and maybe even in your own text messages. The person who sends it or says it is indicating that they're ready to get it on.

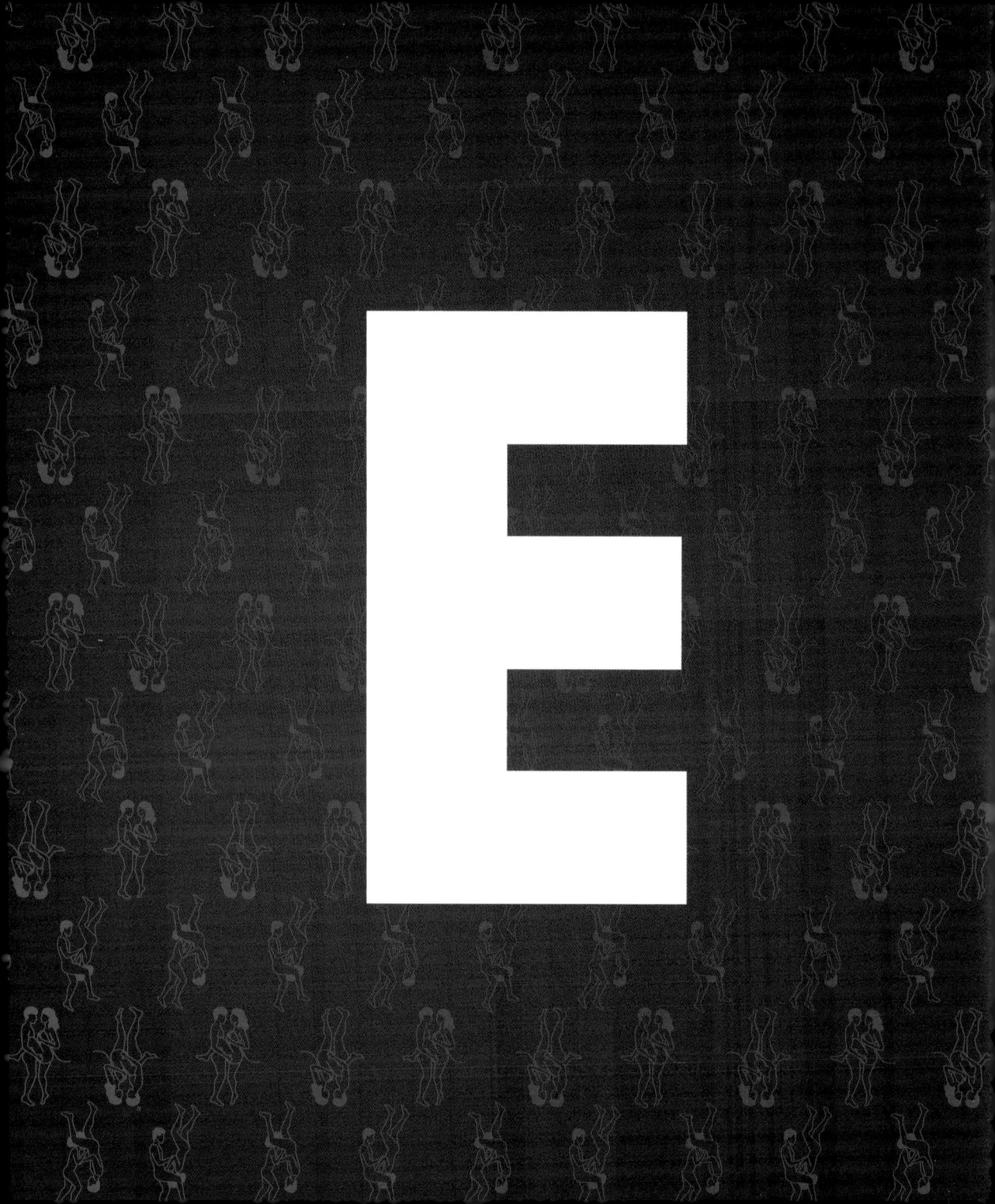

all about **edging**

In most cases, being a tease is just mean. The one time it's anything but? During sex. In fact, teasing out pleasure can lead to an orgasm more over-the-top than a Cardi B verse.

Enter edging, the practice of purposefully building up to and then delaying a climax, so that when you finally do let go, the bliss is extra intense. "It creates anticipation, and when you draw that out, you're able to savor the final moment so much more," explains sex and relationships coach Dawn Serra. Physically, prolonging a release means your body has ample time to direct blood flow to the nerves and muscles in your pelvis and genitals, making those areas supersensitive . . . and your eventual finish feel even more amazing.

Edging also delivers the coveted perk of more time in the sack. One study found that women wish they could tack nearly 8 more minutes onto the average 11 to 13 minutes of foreplay and about 7 more on to the average 7 to 8 minutes of intercourse. And since it takes most guys around 2 to 4 minutes of PnV action to climax and women often at least 10, edging can be a game changer.

Before you attempt to stretch things out, know this: "Edging with a partner is tricky because they need to pause exactly when you need them to," says sex therapist Vanessa Marin, founder of Finishing School, an online orgasm course for women. "Lingering for even a second longer can cause you to orgasm." To get it right, during foreplay, ask your partner to pleasure you down there using their fingers or tongue in a pattern (side-to-side, up-and-down, or circular motions) that feels good. When you sense you're getting close, give a clear verbal signal, like "wait," "stop," or "ohmygodthat'ssogoodbut-pleasehold." A few seconds later, have them start again, but this time with a different movement pattern than before, suggests Serra. (You can return the favor by bringing your S.O. to the brink and back, too.)

Keep up this stop-and-go to reboot and boost your arousal, and when you can't hold out any longer, let your mate bring you all the way to orgasm. Or switch to intercourse, slowing down on thrusting when one of you comes close to peaking, says Marin. The explosive ending will be worth it.

SECRETS OF SOLO EDGING

Start stimulating your clitoris with your fingers or a vibrator (many even have a pulse setting that edges you automatically).

At the same time, speed up your breathing, which raises your heart rate and increases blood flow, says Dawn Serra.

When you feel your orgasm building, back off by taking your hand or toy away, then gently press down on your clitoris with your finger or touch a different hot spot altogether, like your nipples or inner thighs.

After a few seconds, go back at it, then repeat until you can't help but give in and go *ooh* at last!

★ RELATED TERMS:
masturbation, orgasm

ejaculation

It happens when semen shoots out of an erect penis—normally during orgasm. According to Dudley Seth Danoff, MD, in his book *The Ultimate Guide to Male Sexual Health*, here's what's happening behind the scenes.

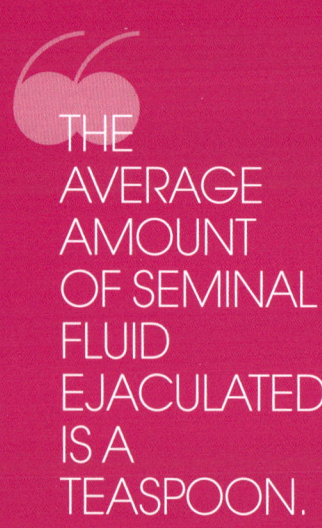

> THE AVERAGE AMOUNT OF SEMINAL FLUID EJACULATED IS A TEASPOON.

- When a man is aroused and grows erect, a pre-ejaculate fluid (aka *precum*) flows from his penis and helps with lubrication.

- Then, when a man is ready to explode, a complex chain of nerve impulses signals the muscles in the pelvic floor to contract, which closes the neck of the bladder and opens the ejaculatory ducts. Sperm and seminal fluid are combined and the pelvic contractions are accompanied by increased heart and breathing rates and muscle contractions in the lower back and abdomen.

- The ejaculate is then propelled from the back of the urethra through the penis and squirts out the tip in several jellylike clumps that quickly liquefy into the opaque fluid we're all familiar with. While the amount of ejaculate varies depending on when he last came and his age (the older a man is, the less he produces), the average amount of seminal fluid ejaculated is a teaspoon.

- Three different organs (the testicles, seminal vesicles, and prostate) contribute to the sticky white ejaculate fluid made up of sperm and seminal fluid (which is used to carry the sperm along to its final destination).

RELATED TERMS: *orgasm, semen*

erection

A boner, or *erection*, occurs when blood flow to the penis is increased, causing it to become hard and engorged. This is typically due to sexual arousal, although hard-ons can happen for other reasons. Here's a few things you might not know about them:

- There are officially three main types of erections: *reflexogenic* (a response to direct physical stimulation or, you know, when he's getting his grind on), *psychogenic* (a brain boner sparked by fantasies or other hot thoughts), and *nocturnal* (nighttime erections).

- When a guy gets turned on, blood flows into the penis at 6 to 8 times the normal rate.

- The average size of a man's boner is 5.57 inches (14.15 cm) long and 4.81 inches (12.2 cm) around, according to a study published in the *Journal of Sexual Medicine*. The smallest penis reported for the survey was 1.57 inches (3.9 cm) long, and the longest was 10.23 inches (26 cm). Girth-wise, the range was from 1.18 inches (3 cm) to 7.48 inches (19 cm).

- Men have about eleven erections a day. Maybe that's why they are such horndogs.

- A man's erection tends to be biggest following oral stimulation.

- It's not you, it's him. Men lose their erections for many reasons, including nervousness, stress, side effects of medication, physiological problems, low testosterone, smoking, and excess weight.

★ **RELATED TERMS:** *hard-on, morning wood, penis*

erotica

Literature or art intended to arouse, these books, stories, and images are usually NSFW. Famous examples include: the Fifty Shades series (duh) and, way back in the 1920s, *Lady Chatterly's Lover* by D. H. Lawrence, which was believed to be so scandalous that it was banned upon publication! How do you know you're reading erotica? If you pick up a book and the characters are doing a hella amount of panting and moaning without much plot, it's a yes. Lucky you!

Q: Are you erotophilic or erotophobic?

A: If you're an *erotophile*, it means you have strong positive feelings about sex. If you're an *erotophobe*, it means you have strong negative feelings about sex. Experts believe that people tend to fall on a continuum between being an extreme erotophile and an extreme erotophobe. We're guessing that, if you're reading this book, your sex game is on point.

eunuch

A *eunuch*, which you may know if you watch *Game of Thrones*, is a man whose sex organs have been removed. Throughout history, according to an article in *Psychology Today* by Robert Martin, PhD, emeritus curator of biological anthropology at the Field Museum in Chicago, *castration* (which can refer to the removal of the testicles, or testicles and penis) has been used with the goal to punish enemies, make slaves more docile, and reduce the urges of sex offenders.

Sure, eunuchs were used as harem guards, but since they were also seen as less likely to stir up unrest, they were used as servants, military commanders, and senior political officials. As recently as the early 1900s in China, castration was a prerequisite for working for the emperor, notes Martin.

✷ RELATED TERMS:
balls, genitalia, penis

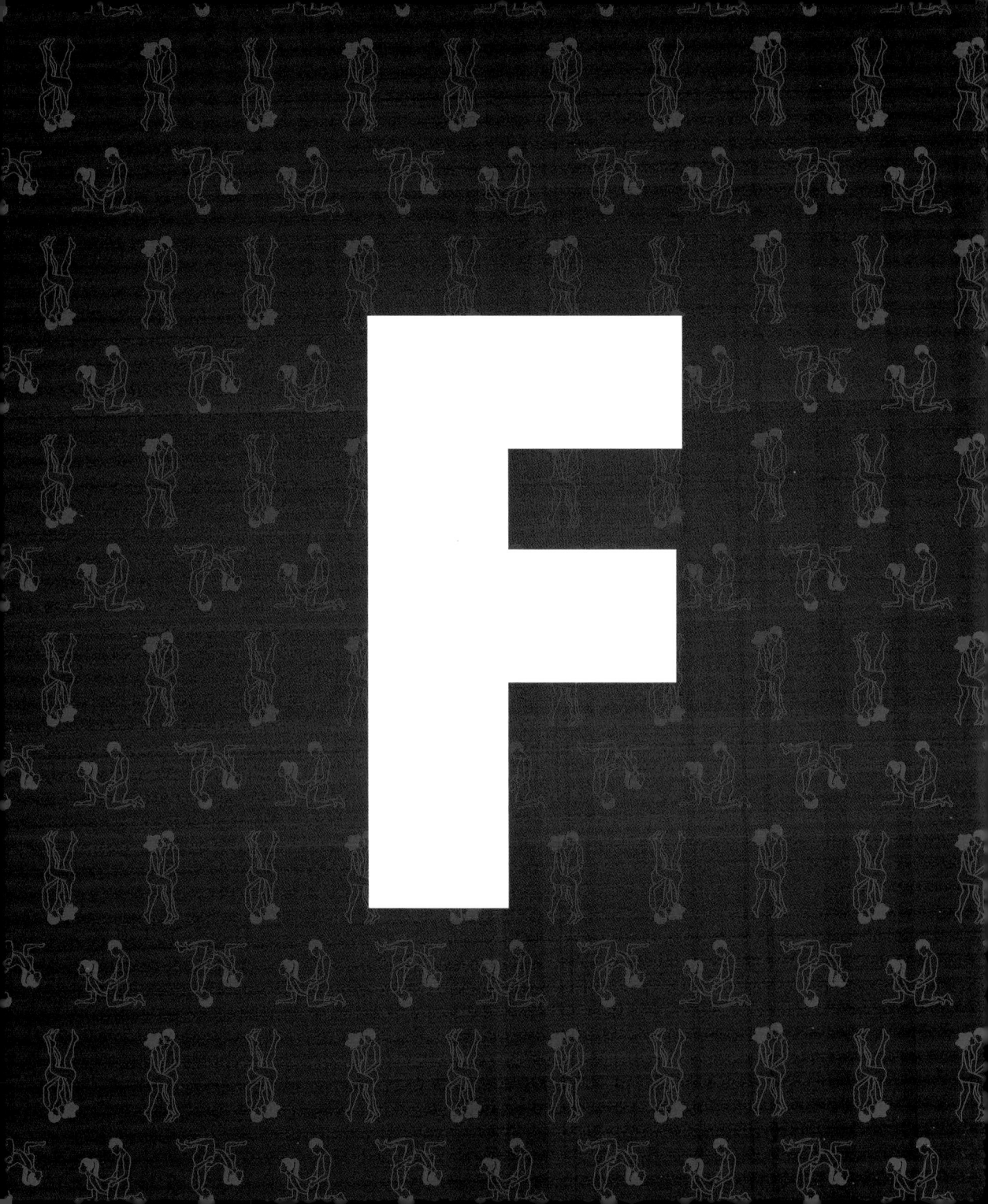

facial

The PG definition of this term, referring to a pore-pinching, lotion-slathering beauty treatment meant to leave your skin glowy AF. But it's also the name given to the sex act in which a man ejaculates semen onto his partner's face. It's become a go-to move in porn, resulting in passionate debates about whether or not it's demeaning. Dan Savage, sex writer and podcaster, simply states, "Facials are degrading—and that's why they're so hot." Others disagree. Real-life couple and sex educators Charlotte Mia Rose and Chris Maxwell Rose address the topic on their podcast, *The Pleasure Mechanics*.

"I think this is rooted in our sex-negative culture," says Charlotte. "If we think about ejaculate as something that's dirty and gross and comes from sinful sex, then yeah, of course it's considered humiliating to have it on your face. But if . . . we think of sperm as a sacred fluid of life, or at least a fluid that comes from pleasurable sex with the person you're choosing to have sex with, then it's a more neutral thing."

Jessica Drake, educator and founder of the *Guide to Wicked Sex*, says that facials can definitely be a submissive act, and while it might not be for everyone, many women enjoy it. However, if the concept of submission makes you uncomfortable, but you still want to try a facial, take control of the situation—and the penis. "If the penis is in your hands and you're stroking it and you are a catalyst

F

for that orgasm, it's a really powerful thing, especially if you're deciding where that cum goes," Drake says. "[During a blow job,] when he's about to come, you can turn your cheek and rest the penis on the side of your face, and then he's coming across your cheek. As long as the penis is in your hand, you're controlling the direction of that cum." You should never be subjected to a surprise facial.

And if you're wondering if there's any truth to the old X-rated wives tale that semen is good for the skin, it's actually not true. In fact, there are occasional hazards that might go along with getting a facial. Dermatologist Doris Day, MD, says that certain skin types aren't necessarily suited to facials. "The water in the semen, as it dries off on your skin, could leave your skin drier," she says. "If you have rosacea, you should be careful." There's also the risk of contracting herpes in your eyes from infected semen, so definitely proceed with closed eyes and a bit of caution.

RELATED TERMS:
blow job, cum shot, ejaculation, fellatio, money shot, oral

---

fellatio

A fancy term for a blow job that comes from the Latin word *fellatus*, meaning "to suck." (Fun fact: A few years ago, there was even a plan to open a Fellatio Café in Geneva, Switzerland, where patrons could get a coffee and blow job for $60, but local authorities wouldn't sign off on it.)

RELATED TERMS: *autofellatio, blow job, oral sex, Z-job*

fetish

When someone experiences intense sexual arousal in response to either "a nonhuman object, a nongenital body part, or a bodily secretion," it's called a *fetish*, explains Justin J. Lehmiller, PhD, in *The Psychology of Human Sexuality*. But simply having a specific preference *doesn't* mean you have a fetish. Say, for example, you really love it when your guy wears tight gym shorts . . . that's not a fetish unless you obsess over those shorts and eventually find that you may need him to wear them just so you can experience sexual pleasure.

TOP 10 COMMON FETISHES INCLUDE:

- Feet/toes
- Stockings, skirts, or other objects worn on the legs
- Footwear
- Underwear
- Bodily fluids
- Hair
- Muscles
- Tattoos and piercings
- Mouth, lips, and/or teeth
- Stethoscopes

RELATED TERMS: *BDSM, foot job, kink, masochist*

fingering

Fingering refers to a person using fingers to stimulate her clitoris or another woman's in order to achieve orgasm. It can also refer to inserting one or more fingers into a woman's vagina to reach the same end, though that will be significantly harder, as most women need clitoral stimulation to achieve orgasm. And hey, it's not just for women: Fingering can also refer to inserting fingers into someone's butthole. Of course, cleanliness is important (especially if moving between the anus and vagina), so wash those hands, people.

When fingering a partner, we suggest using lube and experimenting with the speed, depth, and number of fingers. Fingering can be a nice warm-up before intercourse to get lubrication going. Although popular in foreplay, it can also be a complete sex act by itself.

Some practical advice: Don't just jackhammer with your finger. Alternate between inserting your finger inside the vagina and caressing the clit and vulva. Use gentle, circular motions on the clitoris or lightly tap with your finger. Internally, you can try a beckoning, "come hither" motion with your finger. And just because this is a vagina-centric act doesn't mean you can't involve other parts. Use your free hand to massage the breasts and thighs to intensify the sensation! And, of course, in fingering—like all sexual acts—ask for directions. The best way to find out if your partner is into your moves is to simply ask.

Anal fingering is another fun thing your digits can do, should you be so inclined. Many of the same basics above still apply. It is doubly important to use lube during anal fingering, since the booty hole does not create its own lubrication the way a vagina does. Start by applying gentle pressure to the outer area. Then you can slowly (so. slowly.) insert a finger inside. No need to shove it the whole way in! You can experiment with inserting and removing it in succession or wiggling it around inside. Communicate with your partner throughout so you can both be aware of what's working and what's not.

RELATED TERMS: *anal play, foreplay, lube, masturbation*

fisting

People have very strong feelings on the topic of fisting, which involves (*gulp*) having someone push an entire hand into a vagina or ass. Some put this in the category of extreme sex and consider it something they'd never want to try. Others enjoy it as a regular part of their sexual repertoire.

RELATED TERMS: *BDSM, kink, rough sex*

F

foot job

Similar to hand jobs, foot jobs involve using feet rather than hands to rub and stimulate a man's penis. (It's also great if you want to multitask: You bring your partner to climax with your feet while texting with your hands!) Foot jobs are generally considered an act that men receive, but women can also receive foot jobs, which involves stimulating the vulva and clitoris with the feet. This is definitely a specialty act and maybe not one to start with the first time you're intimate with someone. Best to wait until you know their feelings about feet and everyone's had a pedicure.

Foot worship is another act within the realm of BDSM. A person into foot worship will want to play with feet, be dominated by someone's feet, wash feet, give pedicures, suck feet, handle socks and stockings, etc., depending on the particular type of fetish. In other words, a handy person to have around if you need your shoes polished and cleaned.

★ **RELATED TERMS:** *fetish*, *kink*

foreplay

Kissing, touching, caressing, massaging, licking, spanking, rubbing, humping, and sexting can all amount to foreplay, as it counts as stuff you do before the big event.

As Carol Queen, staff sexologist at the OG online adult toy store Good Vibrations, explains, "Think of foreplay as the activities that are most likely to build up arousal, however they culminate. Sex doesn't have to be a linear experience, starting with a kiss and ending up with intercourse."

There's no right or wrong way when it comes to foreplay. If oral sex is the main attraction, for example, then the touching and rubbing that lead up to it will provide the arousal you may need beforehand. Queen points out that any activity that gets a person "aroused enough to have fun with the other stuff" is foreplay.

SOME CLASSIC FOREPLAY FAVES INCLUDE:

- Nibbling earlobes
- Sucking and biting someone's neck
- Licking and sucking nipples
- French kissing
- Caressing and squeezing breasts

> **SEX DOESN'T HAVE TO BE A LINEAR EXPERIENCE, STARTING WITH A KISS AND ENDING UP WITH INTERCOURSE.**

- Stroking a man's penis
- Sexting
- Stroking a woman's clit
- Licking and kissing an anus
- Lightly caressing someone all over their body
- Fingering a vagina and/or an anus
- Spanking someone's ass
- Playing with testicles

RELATED TERMS: *anal play, blow job, dirty talk, fuck, hand job, nipples, oral sex, sexting, sexual intercourse*

fourchette

This is a kind of decorative female genital piercing, but it's not for all women. A fourchette is the piercing of the piece of skin at the rear rim of the vulva. According to Painful Pleasures, a tattoo and piercing supply and information site, it takes two to three months to heal from the piercing and not every woman has this piece of skin to pierce. Oh, and getting your privates pierced isn't just a recent trend. References to genital piercings date back to the second century.

RELATED TERMS: *genitalia, piercings*

F

Everyone knows that at its most basic, *fuck* is a NSFW (and not safe for lots of other places, too) word for intercourse. Want a glimpse into just how much it's used? A quick Google search shows that there are more than one billion references to "fuck" on the web.

The F-word is of Germanic origin, explains Melissa Mohr, the author of *Holy Sh*t: A Brief History of Swearing*. In an article in the *Huffington Post*, she explains that the term is related to Dutch, German, and Swedish words for "to strike" and "to move back and forth." In the 1500s, it was a popular

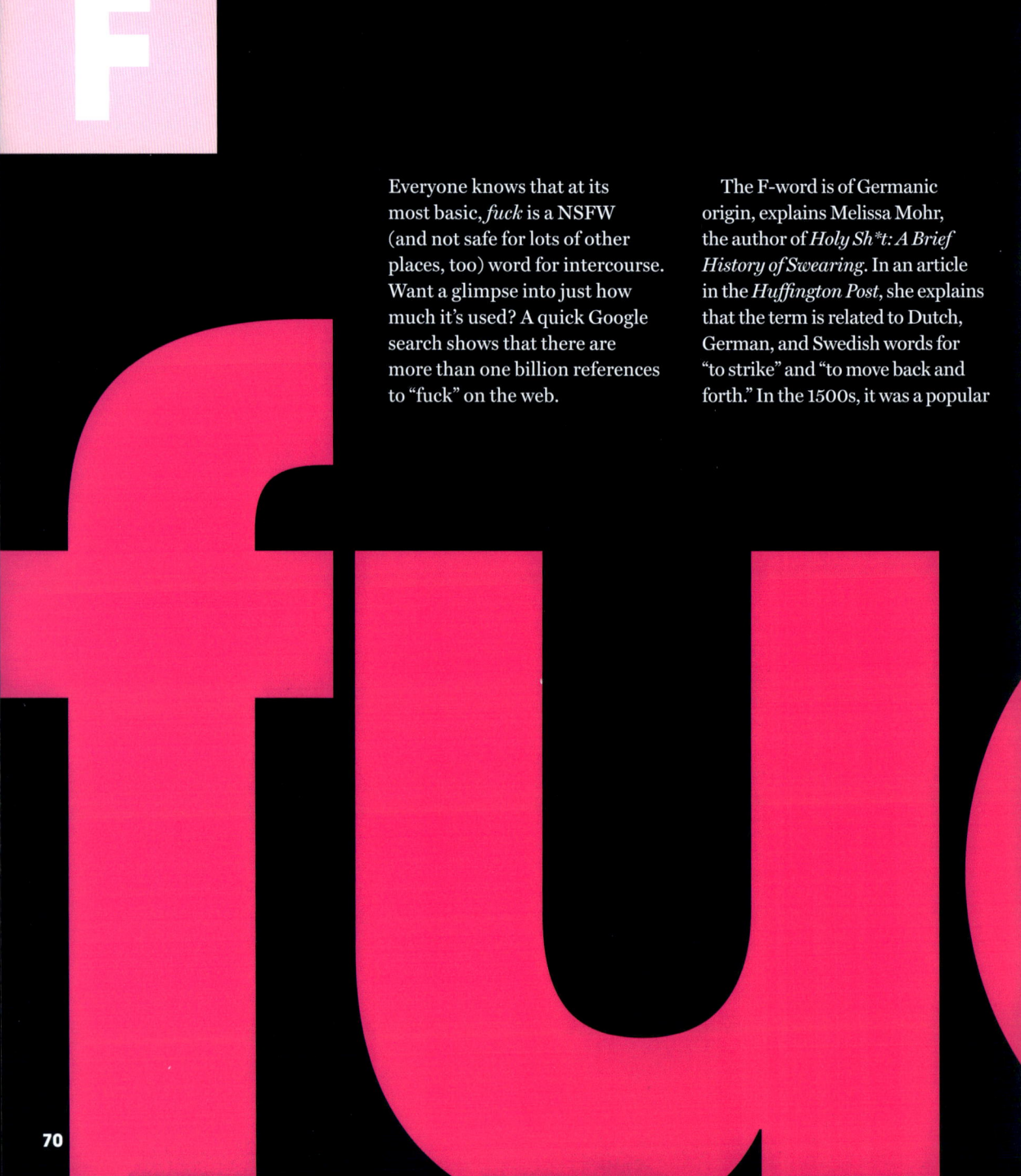

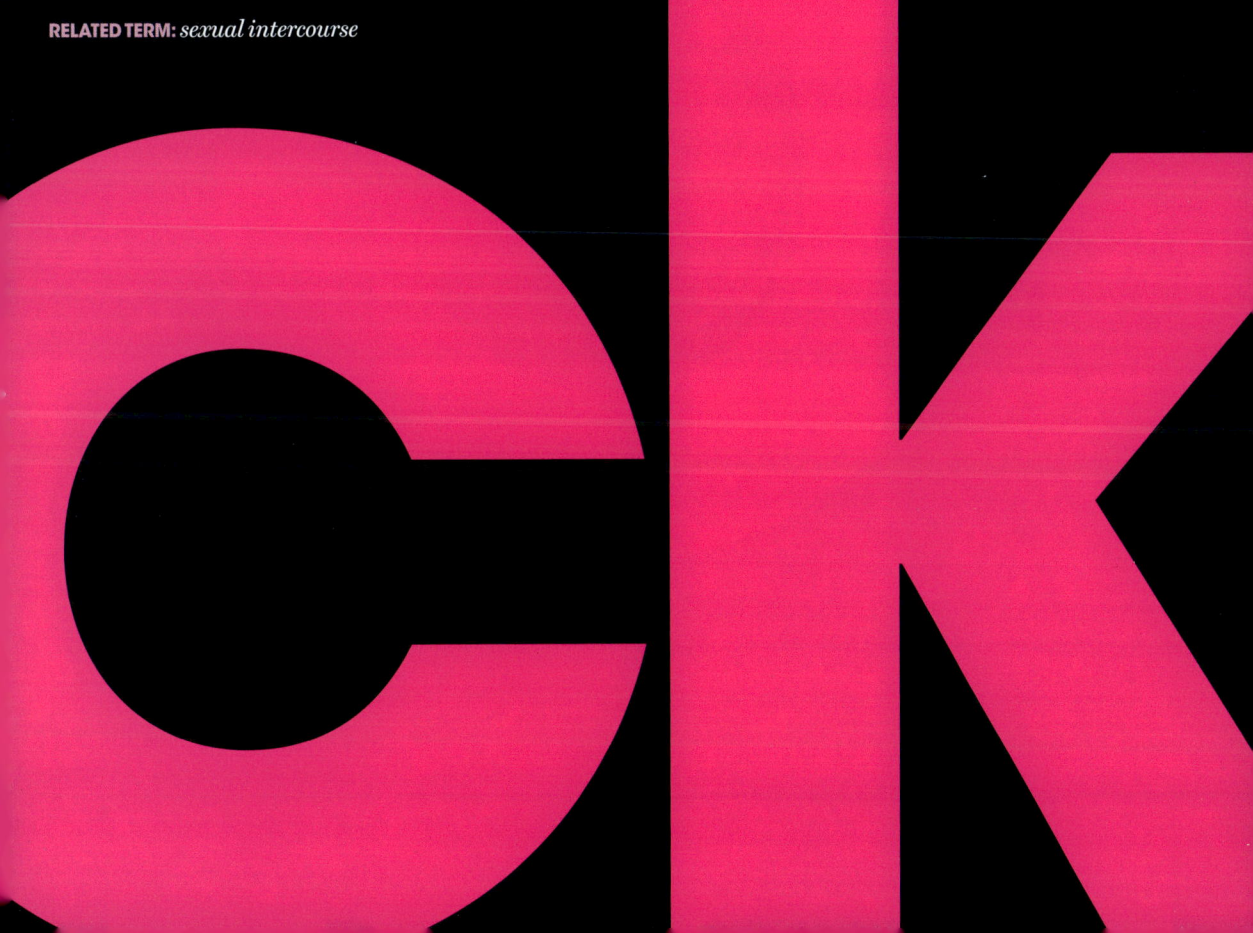

> A QUICK GOOGLE SEARCH SHOWS THAT THERE ARE MORE THAN ONE BILLION REFERENCES TO "FUCK" ON THE WEB.

description for, you know, having sex. But by the mid- to late-1800s, it was being used as an insult as well.

Fast-forward to today, and it's still just an effing great word that's currently used in a variety of ways, such as: "what the fuck," "fuck you," "fucking awesome," and "_____ as fuck" added to almost anything.

RELATED TERM: *sexual intercourse*

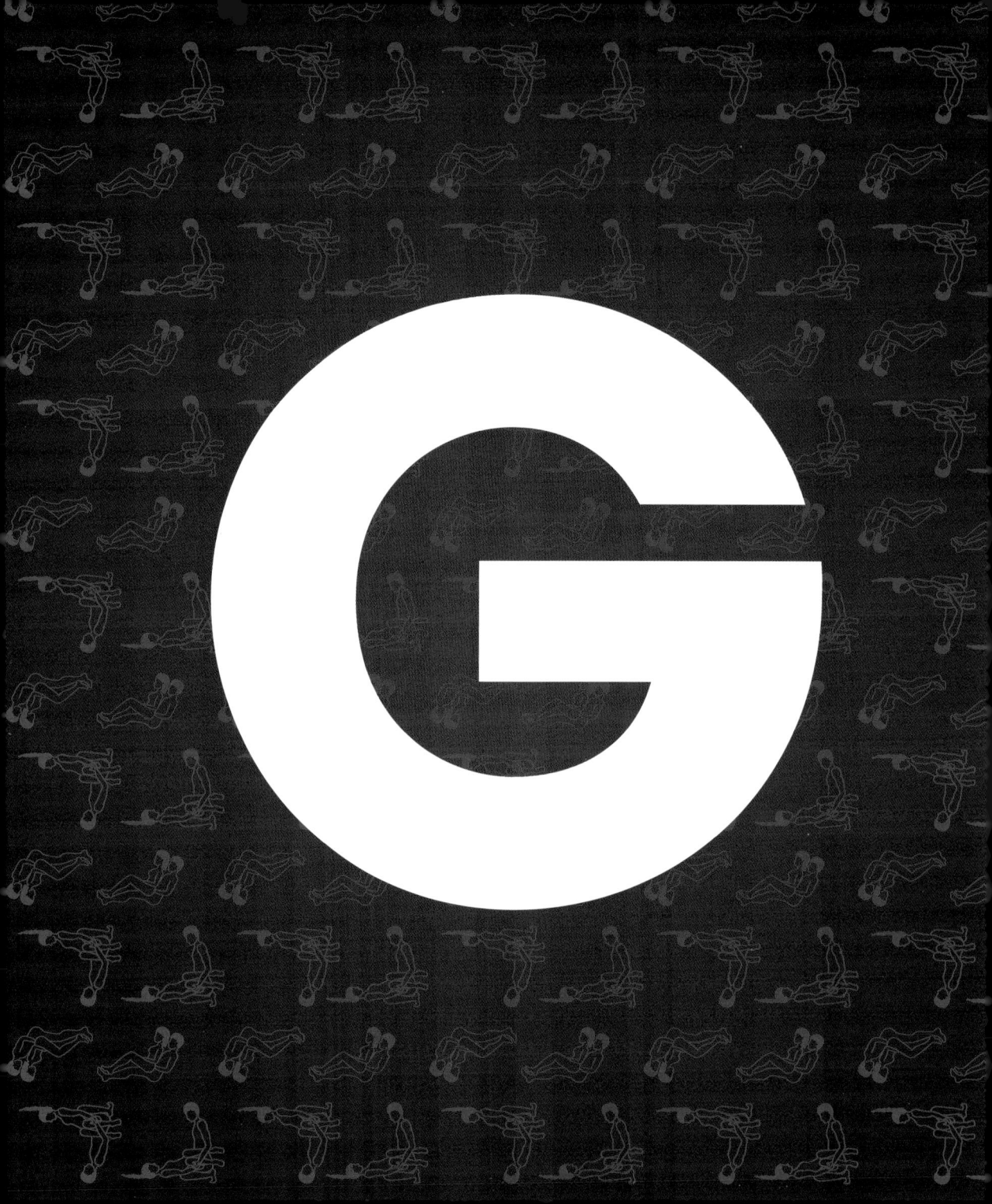

g-spot

Even if you haven't personally experienced its power, you've heard about the G-spot: an erogenous zone located inside the vagina that can produce some pretty intense sensations. Thing is, it can also produce some intense frustration, because it is, for many women, so damn elusive. And though the whole notion of the G-spot is hardly new—sex researchers have touted it for years—the medical establishment has long been skeptical about its existence. There are women and sex experts who swear that stimulating this area on the roof of the vagina can bring incredible pleasure, and there are researchers who swear it doesn't exist.

Whatever the case, if you want to go on an expedition to see if you have your own additional pleasure zone (and, seriously, why not?), here are some ideas that include advice from Barbara Keesling, PhD, author of *The Good Girl's Guide to Bad Girl Sex*, and sex coach Amy Levine, founder of IgniteYourPleasure.com.

- **Try the "gyno" position.**
First, wash your hands. Then prop yourself up on your bed with your legs spread like they would be if you were visiting the gyno. Put lube on your middle finger and insert it into your vagina with your palm facing up. Your G-spot is on the top wall of your vagina halfway between your vaginal opening and cervix. The spot should feel a little rough, yet spongy almost like the surface of a walnut.

- **Get your partner involved.**
Lie in the same position as you would if you were exploring on your own, and prop your back up with a lot of pillows. Have your partner insert their middle finger and curve it back toward themselves once it's inside you. They can also stimulate your clitoris with their thumb at the same time for an added sensation.

- **Take advantage of his curve.**
Every penis is different, but a lot of guys have a slight curve when they're erect. Take advantage of the way your guy curves to try to hit your G-spot. Think: whichever way it curves, you want that angle hitting up against it.

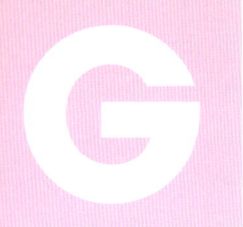

3 g-spot satisfying positions

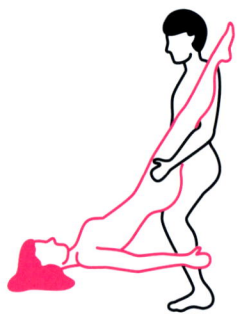

Do the butterfly.
If your man has a pretty straight erection, try to hit your G with the butterfly position. Here's how: Lie on your back on a counter or table. Lift your legs and rest them on his shoulders. Tilt your pelvis upward so that your back forms a straight line angling toward him and your crotches meet. Have him place his hands under your hips so he can hold you close while he thrusts. This position puts his penis right in line with your G-spot.

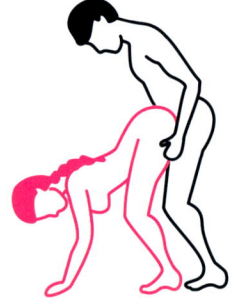

Try it upright.
Stand in front of a wall or mirror with your back to your guy. Have him enter you from behind and slowly thrust in and out. You can experiment with the angle to find out the best way to hit your G.

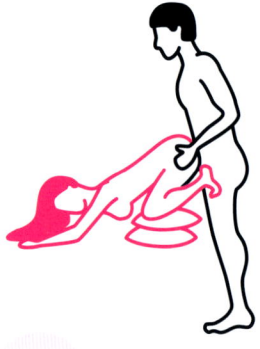

Love doggy style?
Put a few pillows under your knees beforehand—this angles your pelvis in a way that makes it easy for your man to target your G-spot.

✴ **RELATED TERMS:** *foreplay, fuck, positions, sexual intercourse*

gay

It is pretty rare—as in almost never—that you hear anyone use the word *gay* the way its original, centuries-old definition implied: "carefree" or "bright and colorful." In the 1960s, according to the *Oxford Living Dictionary*, *gay* became "the term preferred by homosexual men to describe themselves." It can also, occasionally, be used to refer to lesbians, but in LGBTQA+ terminology, there is a distinction between the two, with the letters generally referring to lesbian, gay, bisexual, trans, queer (or questioning), asexual (or ally), and + for other ways someone might identify.

RELATED TERMS: *androsexuality, asexuality, bisexuality, cisgender, gender, genderqueer, heterosexuality/homosexuality, lesbian, nonbinary, pansexuality, transgender, queer*

gender

We are living in an amazing time when there's more understanding and exploration around the complex reality of gender identity and sexuality that goes beyond the binary options of male or female. Millennials are actively redefining the meaning of gender and sexuality, and throughout *Cosmpolitan Sexopedia*, we take a stab at presenting the most up-to-date terms and definitions as related to gender.

RELATED TERMS: *androsexuality, asexuality, bisexuality, cisgender, gay, genderqueer, heterosexuality/homosexuality, lesbian, nonbinary, pansexuality, transgender, queer*

genderqueer

Basically, *genderqueer* refers to gender identity rather than sexual preference. According to the *Encyclopedia of Gay, Lesbian, Bisexual, Transgender, and Queer Culture*, "The term *genderqueer* began to be commonly used at the turn of the twenty-first century by youth who feel

genitalia

The internal and external reproductive organs. While there are many different terms for the external genitals, it basically includes the male penis and scrotum and female labia minora, labia majora, and clitoris.

The internal genitals include, for males, the epididymis and vas deferens and, for females, the ovaries, fallopian tubes, uterus, cervix, and vagina.

RELATED TERMS: *balls, clitoris, G-spot, labia, penis, vagina, vulva*

GNOC

"Get naked on camera" is the meaning of this sexting abbreviation. Another handy—and bossy—term you might want to use is GYPO, for when you want to tell your partner to "get your pants off."

---

golden shower

The act of one person peeing on another person during sex. It is also known as *watersports*, which is why an Internet image search turns up pictures of people smiling on jet skis as well as people peeing on each other.

RELATED TERMS: *fetish, kink, squirting, watersports*

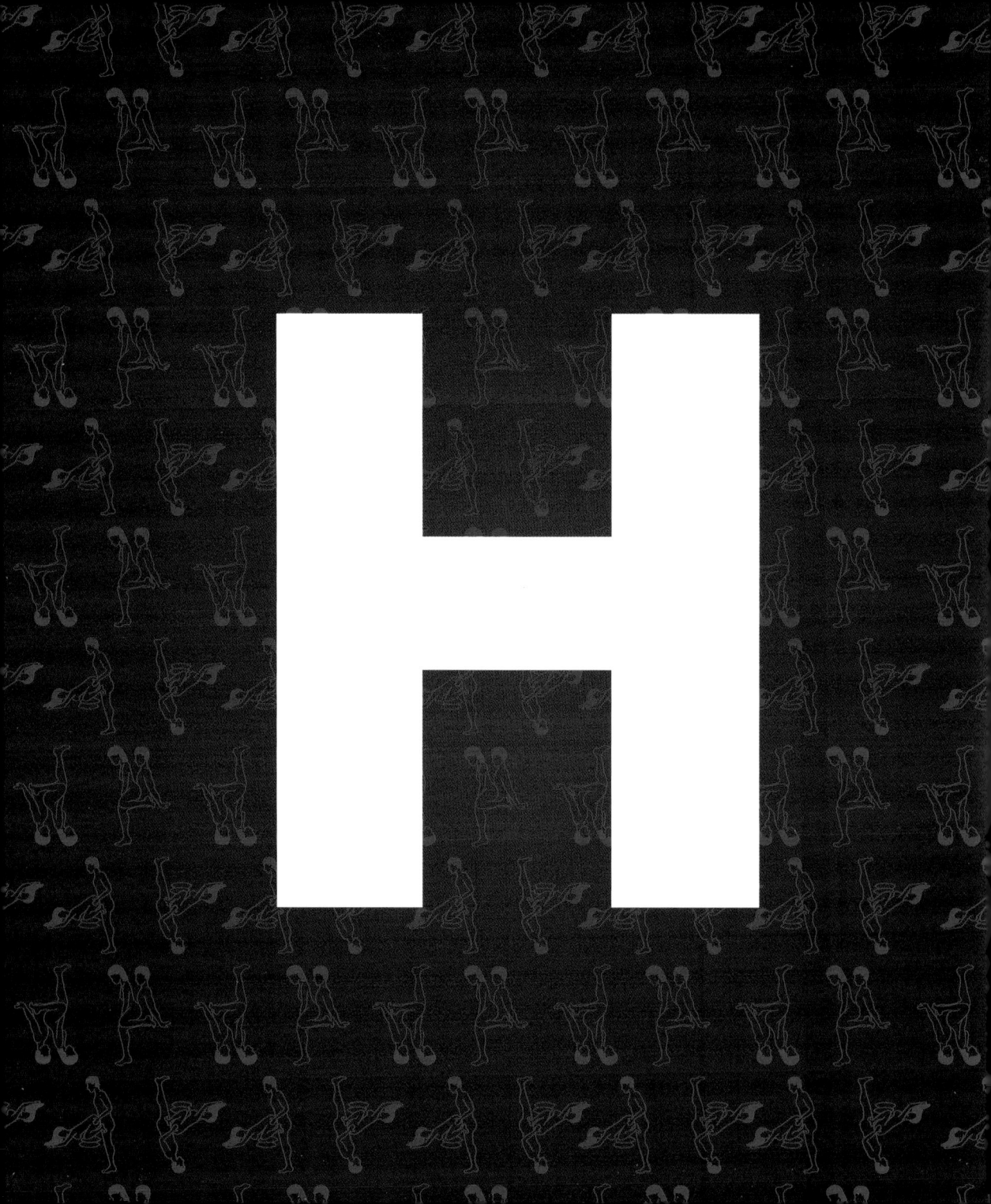

hair removal

Celebrity dermatologist, Robert Anolik, MD, answers key questions about hair removal down-under.

Q: When it comes to ladyscaping, what's better: shaving, waxing, or laser?

"If you're looking for the most lasting treatment, then it's definitely laser. You can wax or shave, but in a matter of days or weeks the hair will return since those treatments don't destroy the hair follicles the way laser treatments do."

Q: Is laser hair removal permanent? And does it remove 100 percent of the hair?

"I can't say that a person will never have to think about hair growing in that area again, since the body is driven to produce hair where it wants. But after a sufficient number of repeated treatments, there will be little to no hair left in the targeted area. Even so, however, it is not uncommon for a person to return once a year for a single session to knock off any residual hair that's returned."

Q: Who's the best candidate for laser hair removal?

"To be a candidate you have to have pigment in the hair, since the laser works by transferring the energy of the light beam to the pigment of the hair follicle. That's why people with light red or very blond and gray hair are more difficult to treat."

Q: Are there any risks to laser treatment down there?

"It's an extraordinarily safe procedure. But even then, the skin can react and pigmentary abnormalities or scarring can occur. That's why it is important to make sure a qualified person is doing the treatment. The laws vary from state-to-state on what services spa-practitioners can perform. Bottom line: A dermatologist or plastic surgeon will be the most qualified. After all, dermatologists are the pioneers in this field who developed the technology. Think about it: Would you have a podiatrist fill a cavity?"

Q: Is it painful?

"The thicker the hair, the more sensitive it is likely to be. Also, keep in mind it's a sensitive part of the body so some areas can hurt and others will be fine. The benefit of going to a doctor is that they can treat you with prescription numbing creams."

Q: Should you ever get a lasering/bikini wax during your period?

"You definitely can. That has no impact on the treatment."

RELATED TERMS:
pubic hair, vulva

hand job

Your guy is the expert when it comes to knowing what feels good in the jerking-his-junk department, but if you wanna help get him off, here's some advice.

To prep for some hands-on loving, don't go straight for the goods. Tease him a little. Run your hands up and down his thighs and lower belly first. Then start stroking the penis with a light touch, wrapping your hand around his shaft, and slowly adding pressure as you move it up and down.

If the hand job goes on for a while, be sure to use lube to prevent chafing (dick chafing = big ouch). To make the motion smoother and easier, Jessica Drake, educator and founder of the *Guide to Wicked Sex*, recommends starting a hand job slowly with one hand, progressing to what she considers her "signature" move: moving the hand up the shaft, then turning it in a polishing motion at the top.

Most importantly, check in with your guy. Ask if he wants you to do anything particular or change up your stroke. Another way to get more intel is to have him jerk off for you. "It's like a private tutorial for you on what gets him off," says Drake.

✱ RELATED TERMS:
foreplay, jerking off, masturbation, orgasm, wank

happy ending

When used in a sexual way, the term has nothing to do with the "awwww . . . so sweet" ending of a rom-com and everything to do with orgasm. The term is commonly used to describe when a man pays for a sexual massage that ends in ejaculation. But women can also have happy-ending massages. Hey, it's only fair! Although, be warned, these sexual massages are frequently illegal in the US—depending on local licensing laws—and not something your local licensed massage therapist would provide.

❋ RELATED TERMS: *ejaculation, hand job, orgasm*

---

hard-on

Another term for an erection, describing the process when a penis hardens during arousal due to increased blood flow to the area. "As a result, the penis not only gets bigger; it gets stiffer and more erect. The action is similar to a fire hose that goes from limp and bendable to hard and rigid as it fills with water," explains Dudley S. Danoff, MD, in *The Ultimate Guide to Male Sexual Health*.

❋ RELATED TERMS: *erection, morning wood, penis*

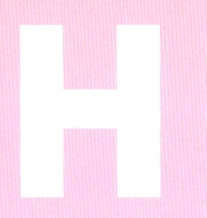

heterosexuality/ homosexuality

"The term *heterosexuality* comes from the Greek affix *hetero*, meaning 'different' or 'other'" according to SexInfo Online, which is affiliated with the University of California, Santa Barbara. "*Heterosexuality* is a sexual orientation in which a person is sexually attracted to people of the opposite sex.

People who identify as heterosexual have emotional, sexual, and romantic relationships with people of the opposite sex. A common term for a person who identifies as heterosexual is 'straight.'"

Sex info online defines *homosexuality* (from the Greek affix *homo*, meaning "same") as "a sexual orientation in which a person, male or female, is sexually attracted to people of the same sex. People who identify as homosexual may have emotional, sexual, and romantic relationships with people of the same sex. Typically, a homosexual male identifies as *gay*, and a homosexual female identifies as *lesbian* or a *gay woman*. Furthermore, someone's identity is independent of their gender identity."

✱ **RELATED TERMS:**
androsexuality, asexuality, bisexuality, cisgender, gay, gender, genderqueer, lesbian, nonbinary, pansexuality, transgender, queer

NOTE
It's important to note that GLAAD now lists *homosexual* in its glossary as a term to avoid because it's considered an outdated clinical label and has been used negatively.

horny

We can feel horny or aroused for a million reasons. It could be the sight of either of the Hemsworth brothers. It could be the result of a little physical friction down there. Or it could be caused by hormones flooding your system, launching the body's built-in "let's make some babies" programming. But once you're really feeling aroused, there are some core physiological things going on, according to the NHS Choices website.

Genital blood vessels dilate and more blood flows into the vaginal walls, sparking lubrication. The external genitals become swollen due to the increased blood supply, and the top of the vagina expands. Pulse and breathing quicken and you may become flushed due to blood vessels dilating, all of which is helping your body prepare to get its groove on.

RELATED TERMS: *amorous, libido*

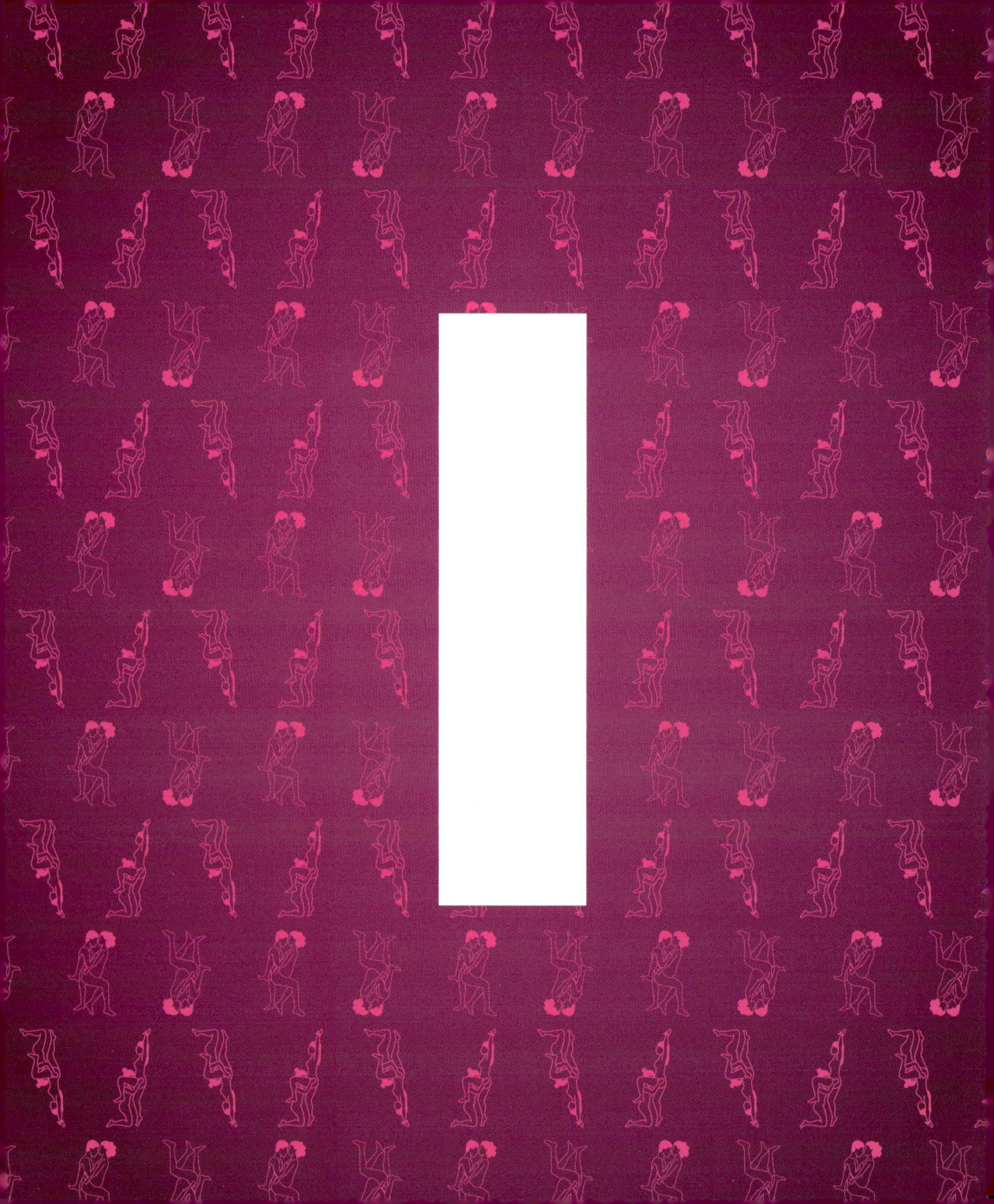

Q: What do i do if my guy suffers from **impotence?**

A: When a man has trouble getting it up, it's likely to freak him out. And even though we should know better, in the moment, lots of women can't help but blame themselves. *Just don't.*

To better understand impotence, we asked Marcelle Pick, OB/GYN, NP, and author of *Is It Me or My Hormones?*, for advice on how to handle his hard-on issues.

- **Think outside the bedroom.**
There are a ton of potential reasons why your guy might be impotent. The issue could be emotional (stress at work), physical (not getting enough exercise), or medicinal (maybe he's on meds that affect his ability to get it up). Even drinking or eating from BPA-ridden plastic containers can cause issues—so once he knows what may be causing it, he'll be better able to resolve the problem.

- **DON'T try to laugh about it, but DO talk about it.**
Since guys generally feel horrible about only rising to half-mast (or not at all), making light of the situation with jokes will only make him feel worse. Your man probably won't want to talk about his nonfunctioning penis with you—but he's gotta. When couples don't talk about impotence, that's when they get into trouble. It's easy for you to start making assumptions, then he feels bad, and you both just end up trying to awkwardly avoid the major elephant in the room. Find a neutral time (i.e., not when you're trying to have sex) to coax him into talking to you about what's going on so you both understand what's happening and how it affects your relationship.

- **Encourage him to see an MD.**
As men age, things like premature ejaculation, erectile dysfunction, and erections that don't last long become more and more common. But no matter your dude's age, you want to encourage him to get to a doctor to figure out what's going on with his D—especially if the issue isn't solved by changing his diet, exercise habits, or decreasing his stress levels.

- **Keep on loving him up.**
Even if you're not having sex (most guys won't want to after they've experienced a moment—or several—of not being able to get it up), make sure you're showing your man affection. Encourage nonsexual behavior like hand-holding, shoulder rubs, and kisses so you can send the message that you're still totally into him, which will help bring back his sex drive and his confidence.

❋ RELATED TERMS:
erection, hard-on, penis

incest

From the very first episode of *Game of Thrones*, viewers were faced with incest—sex between close family members—in (spoiler alert) the icky relationship of twins Cersei and Jaime Lannister. But in all cultures, incest is considered taboo, and in many, it can land you in jail. According to SexInfo Online, which is affiliated with the University of California, Santa Barbara, incestuous marriages are illegal in the US, and in most states, committing incest is a class C felony. However, certain states do not have laws explicitly prohibiting incestuous relationships, as long as the people in the relationship don't attempt to marry. Um . . . not that we recommend it.

intersex

> THE ODDS OF A CHILD BEING BORN WITH ATYPICAL GENITALIA IS 1 IN 1,500 TO 2,000

Intersex "is a general term used for a variety of conditions in which a person is born with reproductive or sexual anatomy that doesn't seem to fit the typical definitions of female or male," according to the Intersex Society of North America (ISNA). The old term for an intersex person was *hermaphrodite*, but that is now considered offensive. It's a biological condition, rather than a condition where a person feels like they've been born into the wrong gender, as transgender people often report.

The odds of a child being born with atypical genitalia is 1 in 1,500 to 2,000, and intersex presents in dozens of different ways, according to a study published by Brown University.

Sometimes an infant is born with ambiguous genitalia—for example, a penis that is much smaller than the norm and could be mistaken for a clitoris. Another way for intersex patients to present is through a chromosomal condition that doesn't manifest itself until puberty, when certain hormones aren't produced. Example: A child could be born genetically male with one X and one Y chromosome, but because their body is unable to respond to certain male sex hormones (called *androgens*), they may have mostly female sex characteristics or signs of both male and female sexual development. According to the ISNA, sometimes a person isn't found to have intersex anatomy until an autopsy is performed after

I

their death, which means they lived their entire life without ever knowing. As for which variations of sexual anatomy count as intersex, the ISNA explains that different people have different answers to that question, since intersex is a socially constructed category that reflects different levels of biological variation.

Upon doctor's recommendations, some parents decide to do surgical procedures at birth. The thinking is that they are "fixing" the issue in infancy, thus sparing their children undue stress during puberty (which is already hella stressful).

The ISNA doesn't advocate performing surgery on a child until that person can establish their own gender identity. They do, however, advocate assigning a child a gender at birth: "In cases of intersex, doctors and parents need to recognize that gender assignment of infants with intersex conditions, as with assignment of any infant, is preliminary. Any child—intersex or not—may decide later in life that she or he was given the wrong gender assignment; but children with certain intersex conditions have significantly higher rates of gender transition than the general population, with or without treatment."

If a patient has all the information about the risks and benefits of surgery and they want to move forward with it, then they absolutely should. However, elective, non-life-threatening surgeries on children who don't have the ability to weigh in or give consent are more problematic. The ISNA encourages parents to hold off on surgery until the child can be involved in the process.

★ **RELATED TERMS:** *gender, transgender*

Q: Do you have **ithyphallophobia?**

A: If you have a fear of seeing, thinking about, or, for you fellas, having an erection, then the answer is yes, at least according to the *Encyclopedia of Phobias, Fears, and Anxieties*. So the even bigger question is, how the hell do you get over it?

If a common therapy for dealing with fears is to give you increasing amounts of exposure to the object or activity that freaks you out, how many hard-ons do you need to see to get past your ithyphallophobia?

✹ RELATED TERMS: *allorgasmia, anorgasmia, erotophilic/erotophobic, zelophobia*

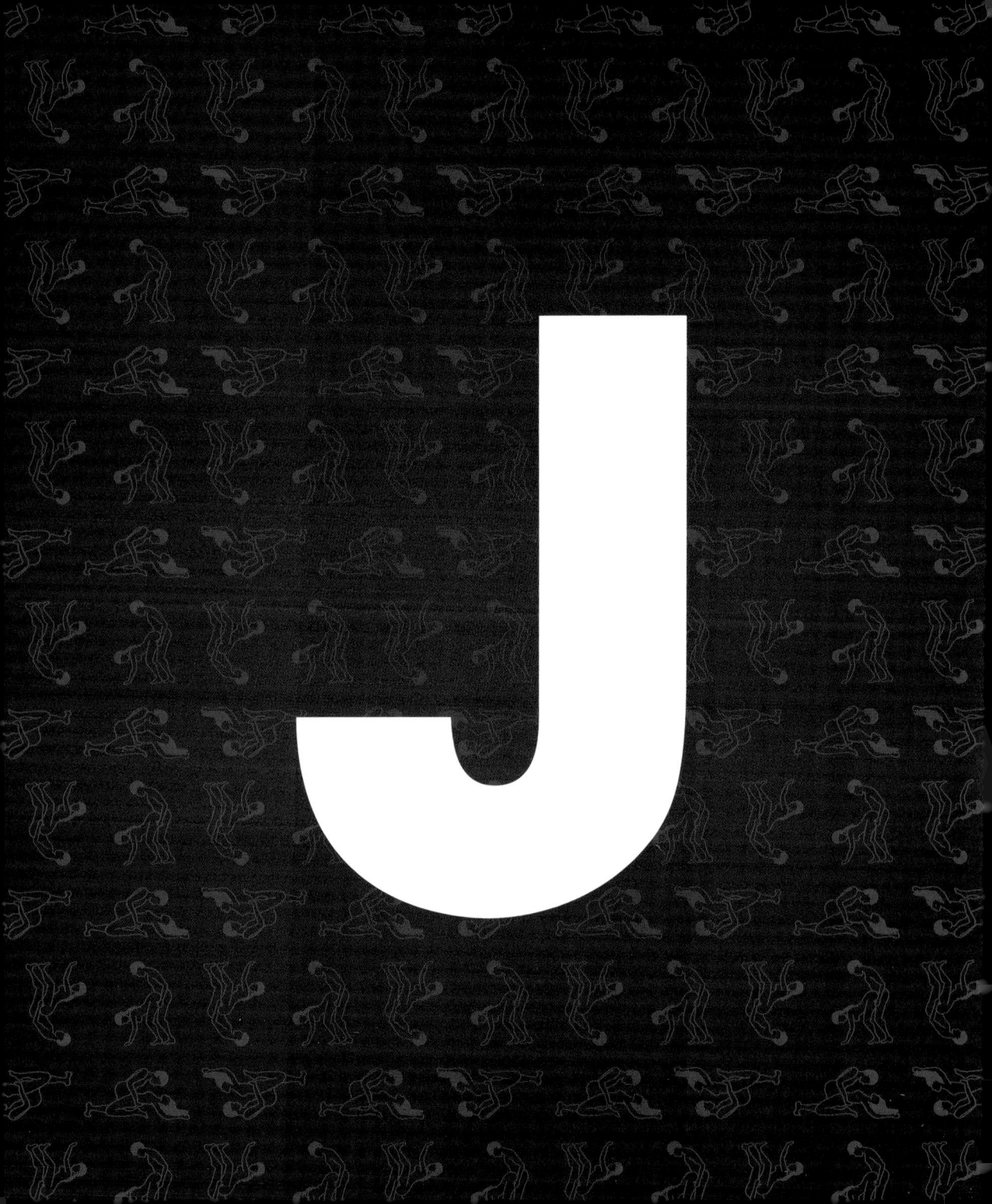

> BELIEVED TO HAVE ITS ROOTS IN THE ANCIENT MIDDLE EAST, JELQING IS SOMETIMES CALLED MILKING, WHICH CONJURES UNWELCOME IMAGES OF MILKING A COW.

jelqing

The practice of stroking a partially erect penis to force blood flow to the tip in an attempt to enlarge length and girth is a hotly debated topic. According to James Kashanian, MD, a urologist at New York–Presbyterian Hospital Cornell, jelqing is a similar concept to using a penis pump. "Penile pumps act by causing negative pressure and drawing blood to the penis," he explains. "They can help men with erectile dysfunction but have never been shown to increase length or girth of the penis." Ditto with jelqing. And there's a good reason to not let your guy try this at home: "If done incorrectly, one can cause damage to the penis, which could result in erectile dysfunction, scarring, or Peyronie's disease," Dr. Kashanian says. (FYI, Peyronie's disease is a curved erection.)

RELATED TERMS: *erection, jerking off, masturbation, wank*

hard answers to crazy questions about jerking off

Masturbation—whacking off, spanking the monkey, etc.—is regularly done by 61 percent of men, if a University of Chicago study is to be believed. (We at *Cosmo* suspect it's waaay higher!) So what do guys actually get up to when they're rubbing one out? We asked Cosmo columnist, Frank Kobula, to tell all.

○ How often do guys do it purely out of boredom?

It happens, and it's definitely easy for most guys to think *I've got some time to kill* and force themselves to be aroused. More likely, though, it happens when we're clicking around online or doing whatever and the mood strikes.

○ Is using a sock actually a thing?

It is. To my knowledge, there hasn't been a study on what percentage of guys actually use one. Most will just finish in a tissue or catch it with their hand. And most of the time, even guys who are coming in a sock or something are still washing them afterward. But not always.

○ Speaking of hands, is the "ghost" hand real? Like, do guys ever sit on their hand until it goes numb in order to have it feel like another person?

Guys have probably tried just about everything when it comes to masturbation techniques, especially when puberty rolls up and drives them insane with hormones. So is it real in that guys have tried it? Definitely. Is it real in the sense that it's a "go-to" technique for a sizable portion of the male population? I can answer this one less confidently, but probably not. There are likely very few people who prefer to masturbate that way.

- **Do guys do it in the shower when we're in the other room?**
Not all the time, but yeah. Guys can have healthy sex lives with you and still masturbate. It just means their sex drive is high.

- **How do guys clean up?**
This varies from guy to guy. Cleanup usually involves just washing our hands off (with soap, hopefully). If we used lotion, it'll pretty much be absorbed by the skin, but with lube we might need to splash some water on our dick. Some will use a tissue, which usually makes cleanup pretty painless. And this is really, really rare, but some guys will even use a condom during the deed . . . no fuss, no muss, but a little odd.

- **Do guys use anything besides their hand?**
Toys like the Fleshlight® definitely sell, though most guys won't admit to using them. But, most guys just use their hand. It's so damn convenient.

- **Do guys think about their S.O. when they masturbate?**
Some guys do, but for most guys this would be a hard "no." It really depends on whether or not masturbating to people they know feels weird to them. Some guys have a tough time using their imaginations and need to rely on inspiration. Although the term is kind of antiquated, *myspaceterbating* is the act of jerking off to someone's social media page, so now you know that can happen.

- **Do guys like to take their time, or do they just hit an orgasm as fast as possible?**
This is another case where every guy is different, but most men can either feel their orgasm creep up on them and follow through, or pace themselves. It's all about speed versus distance and what we're feeling in the moment.

- **Do guys masturbate to porn because that's what they want their sex lives to be like?**
I really hope not. Everyone's been there once or twice (or ninety times) when you're just like, "What the hell did I just masturbate to?" Arousal lowers our inhibitions, and what turns us on also doesn't mean it's necessarily what we want to experience personally. Plus don't forget that most porn is still directed with the viewer in mind, not the pleasure of both participants.

- **Can guys get off without being fully hard?**
Not really, no. You don't always need to have the biggest and best boner you've ever had, but you're not going to be able to rub one out flaccid.

✱ **RELATED TERMS:** *erection, masturbation, orgasm, penis, wank*

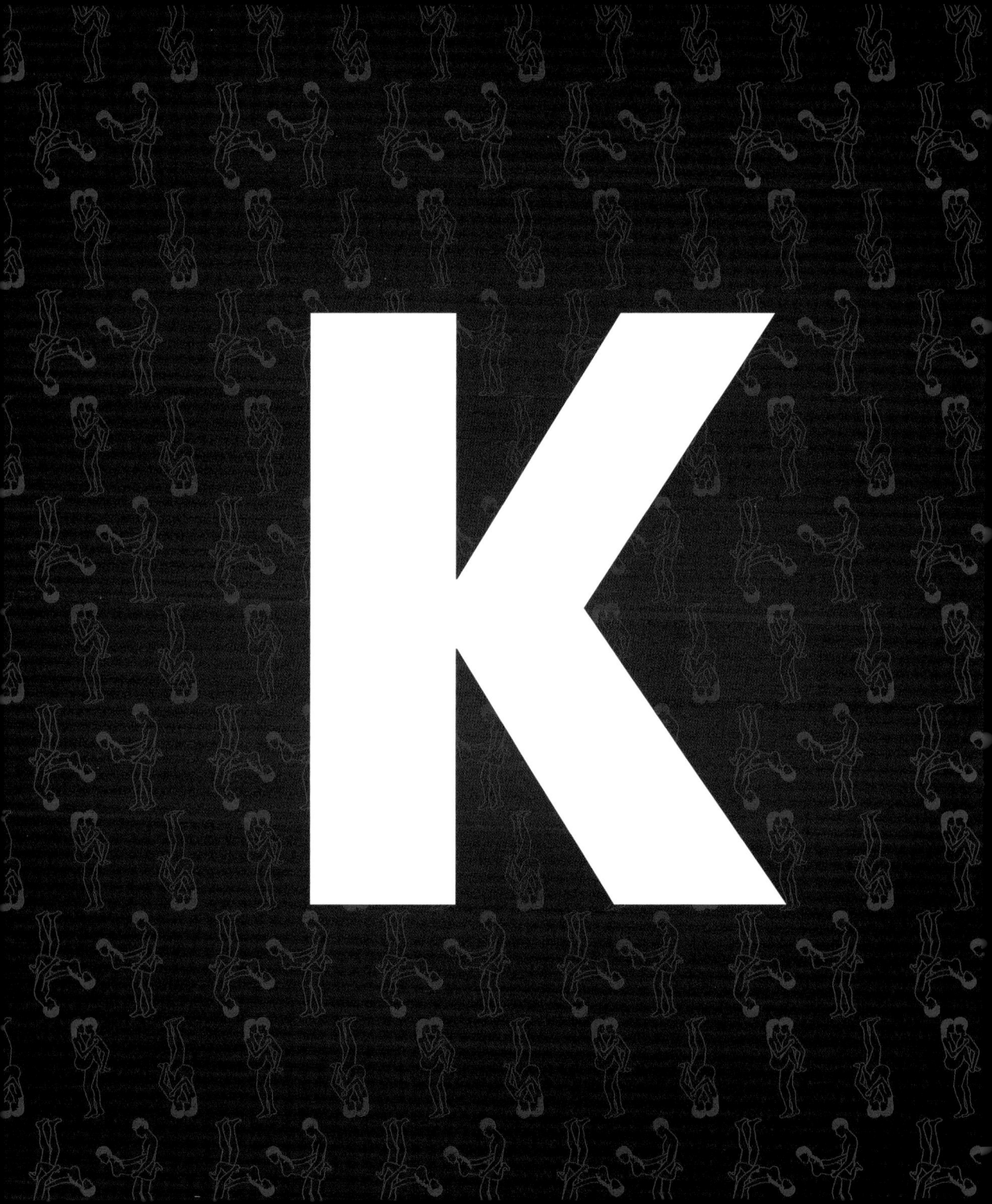

kama sutra

Yeah, you hold in your hands all the essential sex info you need, but way back, there was one bold and badass sex book that started it all: *The Kama Sutra*—the oldest guide to the pleasures and techniques of sex. According to a currently published version of that ancient text, *The Complete Kama Sutra: The First Unabridged Modern Translation of the Classic Indian Text*, the original was compiled in the fourth century AD.

And guess what? *Cosmopolitan* has also done its own versions of the OG guide: *Cosmo Kama Sutra*, which features 99 mind-blowing sexual positions; and the *Cosmo Sexy Sutra*, with 101 epic positions.

RELATED TERMS:
fuck, orgasm, positions, sexual intercourse, tantric sex

kegels

Since forever, sex experts and magazines like *Cosmo* have advised young women to prep their bods for sex by doing these pelvic exercises that tighten the vag. Kegels strengthen your PCs—the pelvic cavity muscles that contract when you climax—so thinking has been that, the better shape they're in, the hotter sex will be, both for you and your partner, since your orgasms will be more powerful and your, er, "grip" even tighter. And while plenty of people still believe practicing Kegels will make sex feel way better, other say they can make sex painful. So the next question is . . .

K

SHOULD YOU QUIT KEGELS?

The down-there squeezing exercises can tighten you up, making sex hotter. But they may be too extra if you also hit the gym on the reg. "Most women in their twenties don't need Kegels unless they're pregnant or just had a baby," says Dr. Rowen. So take note: Doing them just for the hell of it could actually tax your pelvic floor.

IF YOU NEED TO DO KEGELS, TRY THESE:

- **The Quick Hit.** Pretty much exactly what it sounds like, the move requires quick bursts of muscle contractions that work the fibers associated with arousal and urination control, says Melinda Fontaine, DPT, from the Pelvic Health & Rehabilitation Center in California. Do it as fast as you can without relaxing in between. In order to do this, Carol Queen, PhD, co-author of *The Sex & Pleasure Book: Good Vibrations Guide to Great Sex for Everyone*, recommends squeezing the PC muscles as hard as you can, holding for a beat or two, then relaxing fully. If it helps, combine the exercise with a deep breath in and a deep breath out while you concentrate on relaxing. Remember, a muscle is supposed to contract and relax. It is not valuable, and can be bad for you, to concentrate on just tightening. You don't want a strong muscle, per se—you want a flexible one.

- **The endurance test.** Squeezing, lifting your pelvis, and holding for a long time is your best bet for building endurance, says Dr. Fontaine. For a quality contraction, picture pulling up the strings of a hammock as you lift.

- **The bridge.** Dr. Fontaine reveals that "different muscle groups work with the pelvic floor, and so you can get a little extra power by using other muscle groups at the same time." By adding an isolated Kegel exercise to a yoga bridge pose, you're strengthening your pelvic floor and your glutes, both of which play big roles during sex. Win-win.

- **The clamshell.** Another way to combine muscle groups is to do an external rotator, or clamshell-type exercise, which strengthens your lower back and core. Dr. Fontaine instructs patients to complete their isolated Kegel exercises while lifting one knee up and rotating it outward, once again strengthening all different types of muscles that play a role during sex, giving your orgasm an extra *oomph*.

- **The reverser.** Dr. Queen also recommends this variation on the classic Kegel: Instead of simply releasing your PC muscles when you exhale, forcefully breathe out while you forcefully release it. Kind of like you're pushing air out of your throat and vagina.

If you really want to see a difference, Dr. Fontaine recommends treating your Kegel exercises like any other fitness routine. "I think doing thirty at a time would be great... multiple times throughout the day," she says. "Really, if you're trying to strengthen, you can do it as many times as you remember."

✱ **RELATED TERM:** *orgasm*

kink

Depending on who you ask, kink can refer to hardcore BDSM (sex dungeon, anyone?) or any sex-play that's just a little bit more adventurous than standard missionary (think harmless spanking, for example). It's a way of adding some fresh and exciting play into your repertoire.

BTW, a *fetish* is actually different from a *kink*. According to Sandra LaMorgese, PhD, a sex educator and professional dominatrix, in an article in the *Huffington Post*, "Being kinky usually means enhancing sexual intimacy with your partner by adding new and creative elements to sex, such as covering each other in whipped cream and licking it off. In that example, the whipped cream is secondary to the sexual experience that you and your partner create together. In other words, you could have just as much good, kinky fun by wearing *Star Trek* costumes or speaking in different accents. Having a *fetish*, on the other hand, means that you as an individual are sexually aroused by a specific object, body part, or role-play, even without a partner. A person with a fetish might masturbate while they hold, smell, rub, or taste the object, or they might ask their partner to wear it or use it during sex."

IF YOU'RE NOT READY FOR ANYTHING TOO EXTREME, CONSIDER TEST DRIVING SOME OF THESE LIGHTLY KINKY SCENARIOS:

● **Try some invisible bondage.** You don't need tools to bind. Have him command you to hold a position ("put your arms above your head, and don't you dare move them"). Or push his arms behind his back and tell him to keep 'em there—or else. Use your dirty imaginations to decide what the consequences are for disobeying.

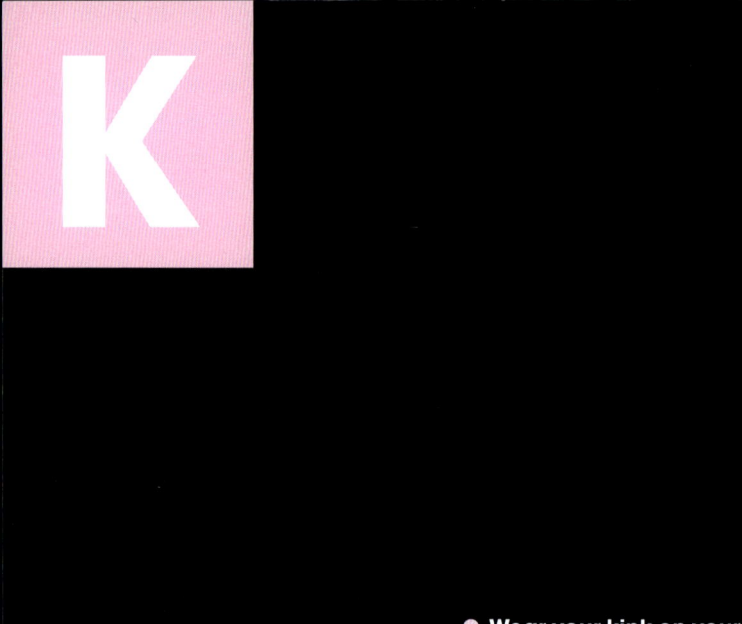

how to talk to your partner about kink

One of the tricky things about exploring your Fifty Shades of kink: figuring out how to get on the same page as your partner. Margaret Corvid, a professional dominatrix, writer, and activist, answers these common questions about getting started.

Q: Why am I so scared to bring up my kinks? Most of us with kinks have disclosed them to a previous partner only to be met with shock or disgust. That experience leads us to approach telling our partners with some nervousness, but unfortunately that [anxiety] can set you up for failure. But, as celebrated advice columnist Dan Savage has often said, coming out about your kinky interests shouldn't be like disclosing a cancer diagnosis. Worries spread easily, particularly to someone who knows you well, so bring up your kinks when you're feeling especially good about yourself.

Q: Are there any rules for how to bring things up? When you're talking about your kinks at first, have the conversation sober, with your clothes on, and when the two of you are not having a raging fight. You should both be in a good mood and have a little bit of time free to discuss this stuff. It's not necessarily a convo you need to schedule in advance, but it's an important one; give it the space, time, and care it deserves.

Q: How do I make my kink more appealing to my partner? Tell your partner the sexiest parts about your kinks—and what they might get out of them. Whether your kink is getting tied up and spanked, or pegging your partner with a strap-on, when you roll it out, you should make your kinks sound as tempting and delightful as you know them to be! Temptation and delight, of course, are a two-way street. When your partner is indulging your kinks, they are also getting something in return—namely, a hot, horny, and responsive you. Kink, fetish, and BDSM are intense, and even someone who doesn't have a longstanding interest can get off on that delicious intensity. Say something like, "When you spank my butt, it turns me into a horny, wet she-devil who's ready to jump on your dick!" That's likely to go down well. Be aware that some people are turned off by kink because their most-hated ex was kinky, or because someone they know had a bad experience. There are also people all over the world who use kink as an excuse for abuse or as a reason to be a selfish lover. Good kink involves thorough negotiation and mutual and informed consent, but lots of people have had experiences with kink practiced badly or unethically. If your partner is once burned, twice shy about kink, talking about how consent works might help them over the hump.

RELATED TERMS: *BDSM, consent, fetish, safe word*

K
kissing

Remember when just making out was the hottest thing ever? Now that you're a grown-ass woman, bringing those everything-but moves back into rotation can help you and your bae channel the crazy butterflies again.

HERE ARE KISSES TO TRY:

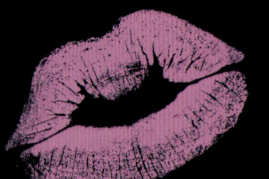

● **The innocent kiss:**
Give him little pecks all over his face—everywhere except the lips. As his excitement grows, trace the outline of his mouth with the tip of your tongue. Move on to open-mouth puckers, but no tongue allowed. If he tries to French you, pull away from him for a minute, then return to kissing. The point is to be playful and work him into a desire-filled frenzy by not giving him exactly what he wants. Yet.

● **The surprise smooch:**
Mid-makeout, suck on his tongue firmly for a quick second. The swiftness will surprise him—you'l practically see the thought bubble above his head saying, *Uh, did tha just happen*?—and the excitemen will make him want s-e-x, like n-o-w.

● **The lip service:**
Vary the intensity and speed of your makeout sesh by playfully

nibbling on his lower lip and tugging it toward you. (Key word here: playfully. Don't bite down!) The little bit of roughness lets him know you're in the mood for an intense romp.

● **The long-soulful kiss:**
Pretend that the only way you can show your desire is with this passionate liplock. Give him a deep French kiss for a couple of minutes, then surprise him by keeping your lips open and pressing them against his—hard—like you want to devour him whole. Then return to the soulful French kissing. Maintain the back-and-forth so he can't guess what's coming. Not knowing what you're going to do next will amp up his excitement even more. You should let him know the passionate pressure is quickly building inside you by switching up your moves and trying something even more erotic. Unlock your lips periodically, and swirl your tongue around his in a circular motion as if you were licking an ice cream cone. He will love that you're in control and essentially taking possession of his entire mouth.

● **The on-the-move kiss:**
Starting at his neck, give him quick fluttery pecks, varying your kisses on your way down to his boxer briefs.

● **The just-because-it's-there kiss:**
If his ears are looking particularly adorable to you, playfully kiss them—it will make the hair on the nape of his neck stand up. Then trace the outline of his ear with the tip of your tongue—bonus points if you whisper all the naughty things you have in store for him. Another fun erogenous zone? His chest. Send chills through his bod by licking around the areolae, gently blowing them dry, and sucking his nipples.

● **The heat-of-the-moment kiss:**
Strip down, and tell him to sit on a chair. Then straddle him so that you are eye to eye. As he focuses on thrusting, take his tongue into your mouth, and very lightly suck on it so your lip action mimics the rhythm of his hips.

● **The I'm-getting-close-to-exploding kiss:**
Softly suck on each other's necks just as you're about to reach your peak. The pressure of your lips against his skin will amplify the buildup you've been feeling inside and create an even more powerful need for that heavenly release. Run your tongue back and forth along the roof of his mouth. This is a place that rarely gets any attention; the more unique the sensation, the more exciting it is for him. Let him know how hungry you are for him by gently biting his back and shoulders, spots on his body that can take a little roughhousing. Place the skin lightly between your teeth and pull; then run your tongue around the area and kiss it. Finally, supersize your orgasm by French kissing him at the same time that you're climaxing.

✱ **RELATED TERMS:**
foreplay, fuck, sexual intercourse

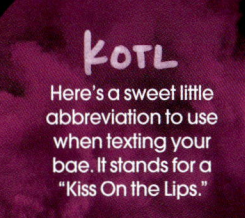

KOTL
Here's a sweet little abbreviation to use when texting your bae. It stands for a "Kiss On the Lips."

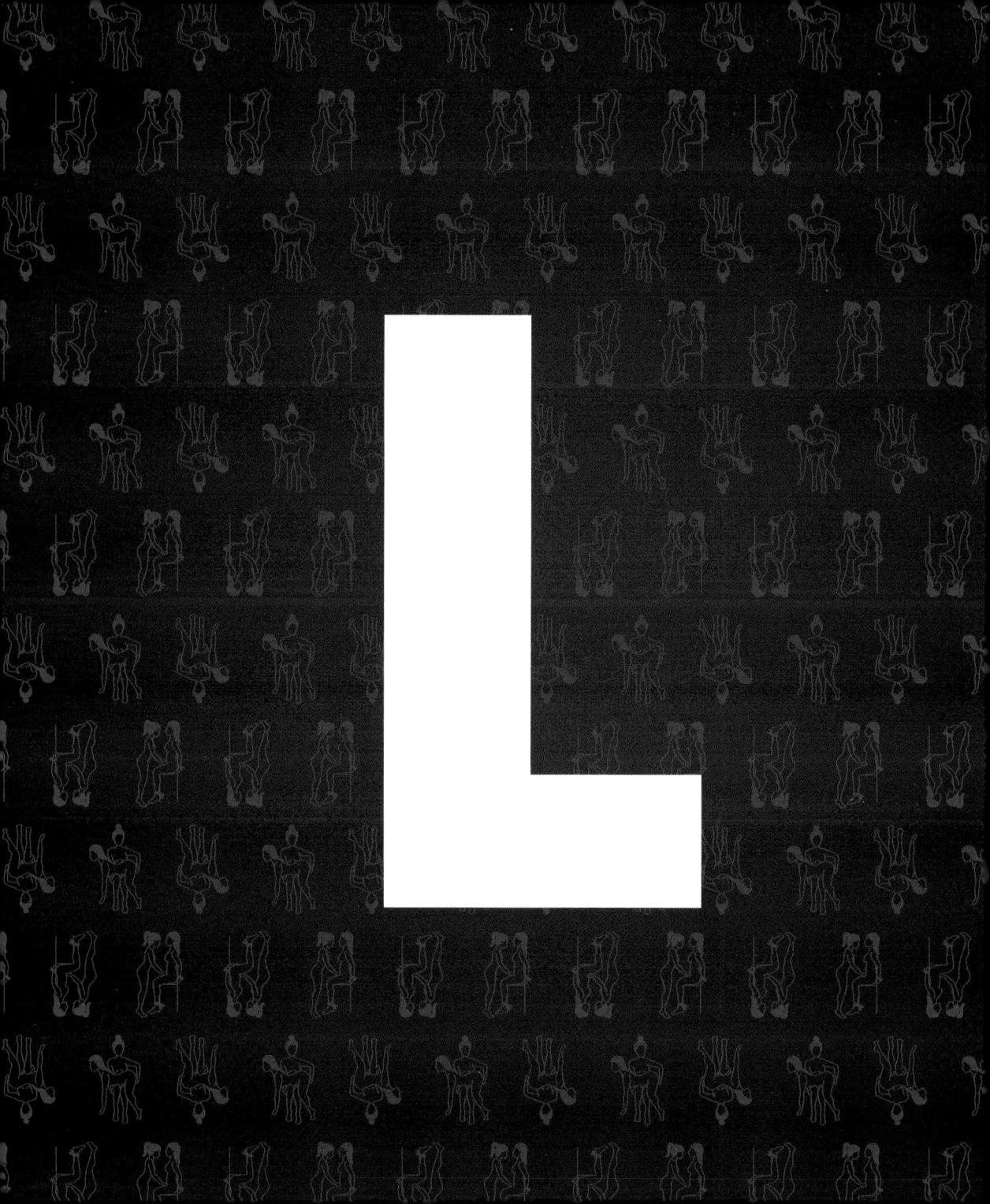

Q: Are my labia normal?

The labia, external parts of female genitalia, are some of the most visible parts of your vulva, but they're still shrouded in mystery for many of us. To clear up a few things, Dr. Levy shares the facts about your majora and minora.

Part of all the labia drama and mystique has to do with the fact that we just don't see as many vulvas out and about as we do penises. And Dr. Levy can back *Cosmo* up on this. "We don't parade around with our body parts like men do, so we're not aware of what everybody looks like," she says. "But as a gynecologist, seeing twenty or thirty bottoms a day for thirty years, I can tell you that there are many variations of normal."

"Normal" is a Big Size Range

Women have two sets of them: the larger, fleshier, hair-covered *labia majora* on the outside, and the smaller, smooth *labia minora* tucked inside. Both sets serve to protect the vagina, both get bigger during sex, and both can vary a lot in size from woman to woman. One study that measured different aspects of the female anatomy found that lengths of (flaccid) labia majora ranged from about 2.76 inches (7 cm) to 4.73 inches (12 cm). The labia minora ranged from 0.79 inches (2 cm) to 3.94 inches (10 cm) in length.

If women were like men who brag about penis size all the time, they'd talk endlessly about their long and elegant 4-inch (10.2-cm) labia.

In some cases, a woman's labia can get stretched longer, to the point of discomfort. One way this could happen is if they're

L

> MANY PEOPLE REFER TO THE LABIA AS LIPS AS THEY RESEMBLE THEM.

continuously getting caught in her clothes. Another example of this, notes Dr. Levy, was an avid cyclist who had damaged her labia after years of long bike rides.

If your labia are uncomfortably long, you can go to a gynecologist and discuss solutions—one of which is cosmetic surgery (labiaplasty). But Dr. Levy says that, in thirty-one years of practicing medicine on about 31,000 patients, she's only considered operating on three women who were experiencing physical discomfort due to elongated labia.

"As a women's activist and feminist, I avoid operating on women for purely cosmetic reasons unless I have a really compelling reason to do so," she explains. "For women who really feel like their lips are getting in the way, I would say that's worth a conversation with a provider. But removal of any of that tissue is removing sexually functional tissue, and it's going to leave a scar that could potentially be painful and may be a long-term problem."

As for the myth that a longer labia, or having a "big vagina," means you've had more sexual partners? That's complete BS. Nothing about your labia is an indicator of sexual history—unless they carry sores from a past STI. And even then, many STIs can be contracted in ways that don't involve sex.

Shape and Color

If you hold a mirror up to your vulva and stare meticulously at your labia (as one does), you'll probably find that both sides don't exactly match. "Just like our faces are asymmetrical, our breasts are asymmetrical, and our feet are asymmetrical, we've got one lip that's a little bigger than the other," Dr. Levy says.

There's also nothing weird about having inner lips that are longer than your outer lips—one study about female genital appearance found that about half of all women have inner lips that are a bit larger than their outer lips.

Although the labia majora are just normal skin, they can vary in color from the rest of your body. Like the inside of your mouth is not the same color as your face, the labia minora can also be a different color than the labia majora.

The only time color can be a sign that something's wrong is if your labia are especially red and sore. For example, wearing clothes that are too tight or rub a lot can basically give you a vulva blister, the same way wearing a pair of tight shoes can give you a foot blister. If that's happening to you, consider switching to some baggier undies and pants for a few days until the irritation goes away.

The Texture

The labia majora skin is basically the same skin as the rest of your body, but with pubic hair on top. Dr. Levy says you can treat that skin as you would any other skin, which means you can use moisturizer if it gets irritated. Just be wary of skin infections like you would anywhere else—especially if you're shaving or waxing.

The texture of your labia can vary a lot, and the only textures that should cause concern are cysts or new moles—call a doctor about those.

More about the Labia Minora

The inner lips do not grow hair and are a bit more sensitive. "Think of the inner lips and the vagina like the inside of your mouth," Dr. Levy says. No, your labia don't have taste buds, but Levy means that your inner labia has the same texture, basically, as the inside of your cheeks. Unlike your mouth, though, the inner labia are lubricated and oily to protect your vagina from any weird invaders, like bacteria and pathogens. And they become really swollen during sex—kind of like a boner for ladies. They also have way more nerve endings than the outer lips and connect to the top of the clitoris, so that's why if you (or a partner) rub your inner lips, it feels so damn good, but rubbing your outer lips can feel kinda meh.

While moisturizing the outer lips is perfectly fine, Dr. Levy says you should avoid putting soap or any other scented product on your labia minora. The number-one thing she sees people with irritated inner lips do is use too much soap. "People are crazy clean—we think we smell bad, or we're trying to clean up all the germs down there, which of course you can never do," she says. "That's the one habit I certainly see in my practice that can cause people to be very irritated." Irritated labia are no fun, especially considering they play such a role in your sex life.

But in case your inner lips do get uncomfortable, Dr. Levy recommends using something mild and unscented, without petroleum in it, that will seal in your body's natural moisture. If you believe your inner lips are infected and they aren't getting better, you should call a doctor.

Your Labia and Age

Since the labia are made of skin, and skin changes as we age, the appearance of your labia changes, too. "Just like faces get narrower and a little bit droopier as people get older, the same things happen to the labia," Dr. Levy says. "But, during sexual activity, they continue to engorge and function perfectly normally."

For a body part that can cause such emotional distress, your labia are pretty simple. And so long as they aren't causing physical discomfort, they're perfectly normal. The odds that you have abnormal labia are incredibly slim. "Anatomically problematic labia are very rare, far under one percent," explains. Dr. Levy. They're just another body part! And all body parts look different from person to person.

✱ **RELATED TERMS:**

clitoris, G-spot, genitalia, hair removal, pubic hair, vagina, vulva

lesbian sex

Lesbian sex = sex that lesbians have, which can include a range of different activities.

The most commonly mentioned lesbian sex term is *scissoring*, which is usually—at least in the world of mainstream hetero porn—two women rubbing their genitals together while interlocking their legs. It looks like it requires some coordination. But according to *Autostraddle*, a feminist LGBTQ blog, the expanded definition can include a woman grinding her genitals on any part of her partner's body. And much like any sexual act, some women love it and some don't. Bottom line: It's not just an act seen in mainstream porn aimed at heterosexual men.

Then there's strap-on sex. According to a recent survey of 13,000 queer women, almost 60 percent have sex with a strap-on. "I love strap-ons, but not everybody does," says Lily Cade, a lesbian porn performer.

"There are plenty of girls who aren't interested. To like a strap-on, you've got to like penetration, [or] you have to like the head game, whatever that is to you." But no, an interest in strap-on play doesn't mean lesbians wish they had a penis. "I don't wish I had a dick at all. I'm so grateful that the dick I have is fake," says Cade.

✱ RELATED TERMS:
dildo, lesbian, oral sex, scissoring

6 nonsexual things that affect your libido

Are you never in the mood? Is your lust engine idling? One of these things could be the reason:

You're hitting the gym way too hard. If your exercise mantra is "push through the pain," then your sex life may suffer. Besides leaving you too tired to hook up, over-exercising can weaken your immune system, mess with your mood, and disrupt your sleep—and "sick, depressed, and exhausted" is the libido-killing trio from hell. If you feel like you're never able to recover from your last workout, you may need to reign it in (especially if your periods are out of whack).

You have an endocrine disorder. Your endocrine system is the network of glands that produce the hormones that regulate your metabolism, reproduction, sexual function, and more. Endocrine disorders, such as polycystic ovary syndrome (PCOS), throw off your hormone balance. Research suggests that PCOS patients face a markedly higher risk of sexual dysfunction (not only in terms of desire but also arousal, lubrication, orgasm, and satisfaction). Patients may also feel insecure about their symptoms, such as acne, uncontrollable weight gain, hairiness, and spot baldness, so they are potentially less likely to want to get it on. It's a totally unfair double whammy, although there are many ways to manage PCOS.

You slouch. The 10 hours and 39 minutes a day we spend slumped over our screens isn't doing our sex lives any favors. One study of 74 people published in the journal *Health Psychology* found that "upright participants reported higher self-esteem,

THE *OXFORD LIVING DICTIONARY* DEFINES *LIBIDO* AS SEXUAL DESIRE.

more arousal, better mood, and lower fear, compared to slumped participants." So better posture could be the sex tip your mother never knew she gave you. It can help us feel more confident, relaxed, and engaged, as well as sleep better and breathe deeper.

You're struggling with a mental-health issue. Anxiety and depression in particular can kill your desire for sex. It can be hard to get psyched about intimacy when you're just trying to get through the day. What's more, many antidepressants reduce libido, not to mention make it harder to get wet and orgasm. Ugh. But that definitely doesn't mean you shouldn't take them if you need them, and some medications have less intense sexual side effects than others. Be sure to talk with your doctor if you are noticing these side effects.

You're stressed and tired. All. The. Time. A study published in the *Journal of Sexual Medicine* surveyed 400 women with clinically low libidos and found that 60 percent named "stress or fatigue" as a reason for their lack of interest in sex, the most commonly cited factor. Stress can make it damn near impossible to focus on sexual sensation, and you don't have to have a medical condition to feel the effects of sleep deprivation on your sex life—too little sleep lowers levels of testosterone. And that's not all—another study published in the *Journal of Sexual Medicine* tracked 171 college women for fourteen days and found that they were 14 percent more likely to have partnered sex for every additional hour of sleep they got. Take that as your excuse to turn the lights off early tonight.

You're dealing with poor body image. In a study of 400 women with low sex drive, 40.8 percent named "dissatisfaction with my physical appearance" as a factor—the second most commonly cited one. Research suggests that women's perceptions of how they look have more to do with their experiences of sex than any of the actual details of weight, size, or physical condition, meaning a therapist's office might be a better place than the gym to pursue a higher sex drive.

✱ **RELATED TERMS:** *amorous, impotence, horny*

L lube

Short for *lubricant*, this slippery substance is the unsung hero of sex. From easing uncomfortable friction to rescuing you when a condom dries up, there's no limit to what it can add. And nope, you do not need to be postmenopausal to worship at the lubrication altar—it is for literally everyone.

Though lubrication can be made from water, oil, petroleum, or silicone, water-based lube is usually your best bet: It's safe to use with condoms, and it's easily washed away (you're at greater risk of getting an infection with silicone-based lube because it isn't water-soluble, so it's more difficult to wash away any lingering bacteria).

If you're prone to yeast infections, use a water-based product made without glycerin; the sugars found in glycerin feed yeast, causing it to multiply.

WHEN TO USE IT:

● **When you masturbate.**
Yes, even sex with yourself can be improved with lube. If you have dry hands, no need to use a moisturizing lotion that could contain unwanted chemicals, especially inside you. Just apply a few drops to your finger before touching yourself for a smoother feel.

● **While using a vibe.**
Imagine the electrifying pulse of your favorite vibrator hitting all the right spots. Now imagine using that same toy to gently glide over your clitoris with the same power but a totally different, more fluid sensation. A dab of lube on a vibrator is a total game-changer. Just be careful: If your sex toy is made of silicone, you'll

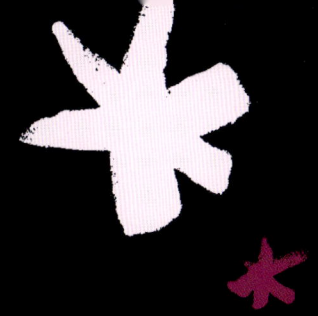
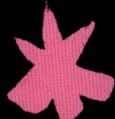

definitely want to use a water-based lube, since silicone lubes can deteriorate soft rubber.

● **During vaginal intercourse.**
There's no wrong way to use lube during intercourse. You can apply it directly to your body, or to the penis or condom itself. Start with a dime-size dollop and work up from there. Sure, you may encounter a point at which it's too much (he's slipping everywhere, it's dripping excessively on the sheets), but that's easily remedied with a paper towel. You don't want to reduce all the friction, but that threshold is personal for everyone and you'll know it when you feel it.

● **Inside a condom.**
First off, no guy should ever whine about how using a condom "ruins sex." But if your partner is looking for more ways to increase feeling while being protected, Eric Garrison, sexologist and author of *Mastering Multiple-Position Sex*, has a suggestion. "Many guys complain that a condom diminishes the sensation. Adding a little lube ups the sensitivity he feels inside the latex." Putting a drop or two inside the rubber before you unroll it might unlock a world of feeling, and it should certainly be enough to shut him up.

● **During anal intercourse.**
While you might hit a limit of "yeah, too much" during vaginal intercourse, that ceiling will be much higher with anal sex, because the booty does not create its own lubricant like a vagina does. Too much is never enough with butt stuff.

● **During a blow job.**
This might sound counterintuitive, but it's true! Sex therapist Gina Ogden, PhD, author of *The Return of Desire*, explains, "Women often use spit, but it can be hard to muster up enough. A flavored lube provides enough wetness that your jaw won't get as tired." So there you have it.

● **For a sexy massage.**
Since any good-quality lube is body-safe, why not try it during nonsexual foreplay? Using it to aid a back massage can take things from relaxing to "holy hell your touch is electrifying, can we please have sex?"

✱ **RELATED TERMS:**
anal, anal play, fuck, masturbation, orgasm, sex toys, sexual intercourse

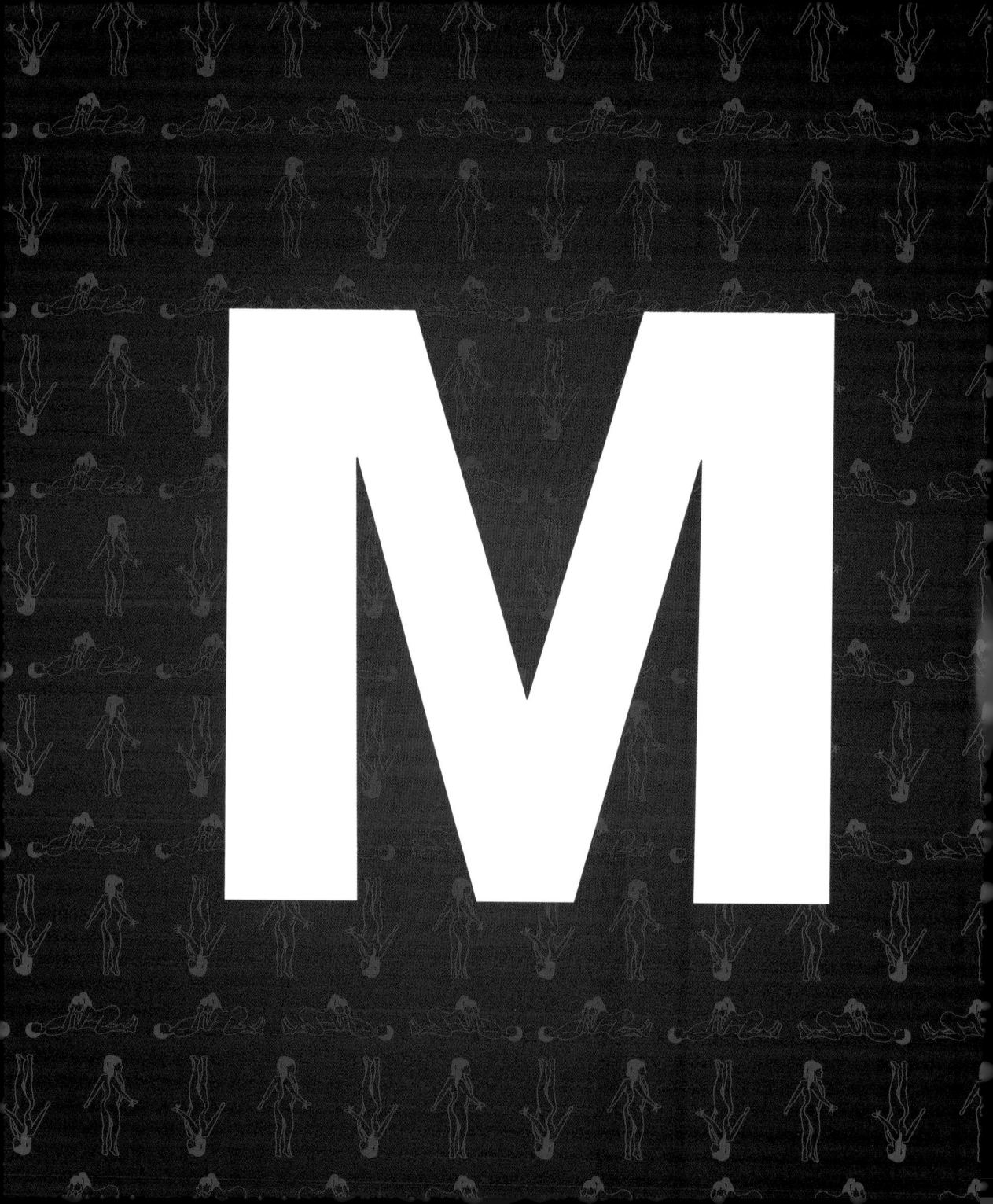

Cosmo's Guide to his m-zone

When it comes to pleasing themselves, men head straight for their Ds. (Hey, it's easy access.) But when your guy's in your hands, it pays to take a circuitous path to his package. We call this the M-zone, which represents the letter *M* shape you make on his body when you touch him in this ultrasensitive, nerve-packed terrain between his upper thighs and lower stomach. Here's what we suggest:

Tantalize his thighs.
Have him lie down on his back on a comfy bed with his legs spread about 6 inches apart. Either kneel beside his bod or gently straddle him, sitting back on his lower thighs. Rub your hands together to warm them up (you can also use a bit of massage or warming oil), then rest them palm down on each of his upper thighs. Just go slowly. Knead him on the outside of his thigh only, and with light contact at first, gradually build up to the point where you're using considerable pressure (like when you're smoothing creases out of a shirt).

Slowly move up and down and side to side over this outer upper-thigh area, mixing up your moves between long, smooth strokes and circular kneading motions. Don't be afraid of getting too rough, since these muscles—his quads—are usually among his strongest and thickest. Switch to softer, lighter feathering motions as you move closer to his inner thighs, where the nerve endings become finer. He will be extra sensitive there and can be stimulated by the slightest stroke.

Slide up to his hip bones. Move your hands upward toward his hips without ever lifting them off his body, stopping right above and inside the hip bones—never putting any pressure on his bones but just making gentle circles with the tips of your fingers, then switching to light swirling motions with your tongue.

Arouse his "almost" area.
All it takes is a light touch to stimulate this lava-hot region. Slide your fingers diagonally inward, way below his belly button, just above where his lower abs end and his pubic hair starts. Take your time and try blowing on the area lightly, segueing into long sensual licks—and if he's not ultrasensitive, nibbling—across this smooth stretch of skin. He will expect you to go straight to his D, so by making him wait, the sex will be more potentially pleasurable.

✱ **RELATED TERMS:**
balls, genitalia, penis, pubic hair

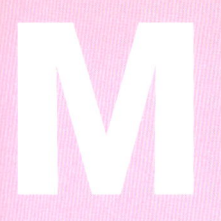

masochist

If you've ever fantasized about getting spanked, you may think you understand masochism, but it's actually more complex than you think.

ACCORDING TO PSYCHOLOGIST NEEL BURTON, MD, HERE ARE FEW THINGS TO KNOW:

- Taking on a role of subjugation and helplessness can offer a release from stress, the burden of responsibility, or guilt. It can also evoke feelings of dependency, safety, and protection, which can serve as a proxy for intimacy.

- The masochist may derive pleasure from earning the approval of the sadist, commanding his full attention, and, in a sense, controlling him.

- While sadomasochists seek out pain and humiliation in the context of love and sex, they do not do so in other situations and dislike simple, unfettered violence or abuse as much as the next person.

RELATED TERMS:
BDSM, fetish, kink, safe word

> "GETTING YOURSELF OFF IS A HEALTHY (AND, HI, ORGASMIC) PART OF YOUR SELF-CARE REGIMEN THAT COMES WITH A TON OF DOES-A-BODY-GOOD PERKS.

masturbation

Pleasuring yourself reduces your stress levels and elevates your mood, says sex therapist Kat Van Kirk, PhD. It also encourages more positive feelings toward yourself and your body. Jackpot! Some 85 percent of women ages 18 to 34 already pleasure themselves, and 35 percent of those do so several times a week, according to a 2017 Skyn® Condoms millennial sex survey.

If you've never tried it, masturbating is a great way to figure out what you like and what feels good, without any pressure or risk of pregnancy or STIs. Also, seriously, orgasms.

The first thing to do is get a mirror and take a look at what's between your legs. Then touch yourself. Most women require direct—or close-to-direct—stimulation of the clitoris to orgasm. Usually inserting something into the vagina isn't enough, despite what TV, movies, and porn show us. (Honestly, never use porn to learn about real-world sex.)

Women report using all sorts of things to masturbate: vibrators, common household items like hairbrushes, and even rubbing up against the corners of furniture or pillows. Your whole house is a potential treasure trove of orgasms!

A FEW EASY TECHNIQUES TO START WITH:

○ **Start with your fingers.** Wash your hands, then try taking your pointer or middle fingers and moving them in gentle circles on your clitoris. You might also enjoy a soft tapping motion. Jackhammering your fingers inside yourself isn't likely to feel great, although some women do prefer internal stimulation. With your free hand, feel free to touch your breasts or play with your nipples. Also, use lube! Having a slick surface can prevent chafing or irritation, plus it just feels good. Bottom line: Take your time and explore all parts of your vag—clit, vulva, and inside your vagina. The best part is that you're in control . . . so experiment!

○ **Use a vibe.** While some women enjoy masturbating by using their fingers to stimulate themselves, many women prefer using vibrators. There is no right or wrong way to masturbate; it's all about your preference. Some might find the buzzing of a sex toy directly on their clitoris too intense, but for others, it's a recipe for maximum bliss.

○ **Mutual masturbation.** Exactly what it sounds like, this partnered sex act involves two people masturbating in front of each other. The easiest way to do it is lying next to each other on a bed. Mutual masturbation might feel embarrassing or way too vulnerable, but it can be educational and helpful. What better way to learn how to get your partner off than watching them do it in front of you?

★ **RELATED TERMS:** *autofellatio, fingering, jerking off, lube, orgasm, sex toys, vibrators*

M

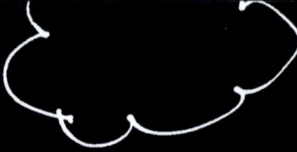

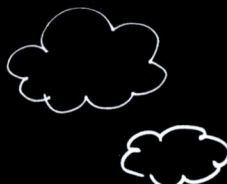

mile-high club

For lots of people, a plane ride means time to zone out. Then there are *waaay* more adventurous travelers who view a flight as an opportunity to, well, bang one out in the teeny airplane bathroom. Since these erotic escapades take place in the sky, anyone who has sex on a plane in flight is considered a member of this elite union. According to a delightful—and slightly worrying—history published in *The Atlantic*, the first member of the mile-high club was Lawrence Burst Sperry, the guy who invented autopilot.

While some people might try to "do it" on the DL in their seats, the most common place to bone is in the bathroom. But it's risky, since depending on where you are, you could get arrested for having sex in public. For instance, one set of strangers on a plane flying from Los Angeles to Detroit apparently felt a sexy connection. So much so that she proceeded to give him a blow job at their seats. They were caught by the flight attendant, arrested upon landing, and faced felony charges by the FBI. Bottom line: If you're tempted to join the club be careful not to get caught!

RELATED TERMS:
fuck, kink, sexual intercourse

MILF

In case you had any doubt, people really dig mature and experienced women. According to PornHub, in 2017, MILF—which stands for "mom I'd like to fuck"—was the site's third-most-popular search term in the ENTIRE WORLD. And after "lesbian," it was the video category with the most views.

missionary

Although haters might consider the missionary sex position vanilla, it's a go-to classic for a reason. When you're rocking the mish posish, the woman has the option of doing practically nothing. You just lie back and enjoy the ride while the man burns calories doing sexual Pilates, trying to get you off. What's not to love?

Another great thing that this position has going for it: There's a ton of skin-to-skin contact. Considered one of the more "romantic" positions, missionary enables you to kiss, caress, and look into your partner's eyes. No one really knows for certain why it's called "missionary," but a popular myth is that the name came from European missionaries who were trying to teach it to the people they were colonizing. According to the *Reader's Digest Guide to Love & Sex*, "The missionary position is so called because it was allegedly the sexual position recommended by Christian missionaries to their Polynesian converts in the era of European colonialism." (Talk about micromanaging.)

This position isn't just for the lazy divas of the world. It's also great for nervous newbies, because it's really simple to do. The way it works for a heterosexual couple, the woman lies on her back with her legs spread open while the man lies on top, facing her. The dude generally controls the power and depth of thrusting while the

HEAT IT UP!

Step up your game with this sexy tweak.

Assume standard missionary, but have your partner shift up a bit so that their hips are higher than yours. Once they're inside you, have them lift their hips to grind their pubic bone against your clitoris. Whether they circle around, rub up and down, or sway side-to-side doesn't matter as long as it feels amazing. When you're getting close, wrap your legs around their butt and pull them in for a deep, long kiss. Who knows? You may even achieve the most romantic sex feat—the simultaneous O!

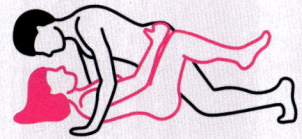

M

> MISSIONARY IS NOT JUST ABOUT A CALM, QUIET POSITION. IT CAN GET PRETTY ROLLICKING.

woman can move her hips and grind. As the bottom, you have choices. During some sex sessions, you might want to lie back with vacation arms and enjoy the view, and other days, you might want to be more involved, kissing, touching, and grinding your partner.

One way to mix up missionary: Change up the position of your legs, "such as the person on the bottom putting their legs over the arms of the person above, which opens up the vulvovaginal area a lot. Even more so if you put your legs over the shoulders," says Carol Queen, staff sexologist at online sex-toy store Good Vibrations.

"Missionary is not just about a calm, quiet position. It can get pretty rollicking."

This position can also be used in anal sex in gay relationships. In this pairing, the bottom partner lifts his legs and draws his knees to his chest while the man on top aligns his penis with the anus for penetration. Lesbian couples can also rub vulvas against each other or use vibrators, sex toys, or hands to penetrate each other in this position.

RELATED TERMS: *anal, fuck, lesbian sex, positions, sexual intercourse*

money shot

In porn, the *money shot* is the scene that shows a man ejaculating in all his messy glory. But, according to an article on Vulture.com, the term was first used to describe the most expensive filming sequence in a movie (which is often filming another kind of big explosion!).

RELATED TERMS: *ejaculation, orgasm*

monogamy

When two people are sexually exclusive with each other during the time they are together as a couple.

RELATED TERMS: *consensual nonmonogamy*

---

morning-after pill

Probably the most well-known form of emergency contraception, Plan B One-Step® (as well as other generic, progestin-only emergency-contraceptive pills) is a single-dose pill you can take after unprotected sex to prevent pregnancy. It's about 95-percent effective within the first 24 hours and about 88-percent effective, on average, within 72 hours. Plan B and other progestin-only pills decrease in effectiveness for people who are obese or have a BMI greater than 35. It works by interfering with egg transport, initially blocking ovulation, or interfering with the implantation of a fertilized egg.

RELATED TERMS: *condoms, fuck, sexual intercourse, withdrawal*

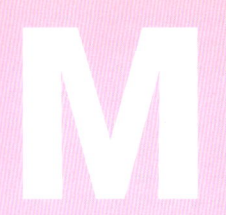

morning wood

Another name for a *sleep erection* or *nocturnal penile tumescence*—yeah, we know that last one sounds kinda freaky. These nonsexual erections happen to all healthy men and, explains Dudley S. Danoff, MD, in *The Ultimate Guide to Male Sexual Health*, "each episode lasts about half an hour, although the penis is not fully erect the entire time. Regardless of age, men get these nocturnal erections three to five times a night. They occur in cycles, separated by one to two hours. Most coincide with the REM (rapid eye movement) stage of sleep, the period in which dreaming occurs."

So it's probably not his fault if his D comes knocking up against you when you're sleeping, and it doesn't necessarily mean that he's desperate for a sex sesh.

🌸 **RELATED TERMS:** *erection, hard-on, penis, wet dream*

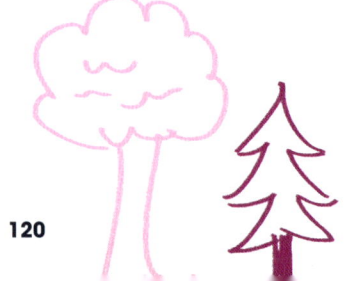

Q: What is motorboating?

A: This has nothing to do with active, high-speed watersports, though it probably burns a few calories. Motorboating is the act of putting your face in between someone's breasts and moving your head back and forth quickly while making a raspberry sound with your tongue and lips. While the act can skew jokey, for some, it's a real turn-on.

❋ RELATED TERMS: *breasts, fetish, foreplay, kink*

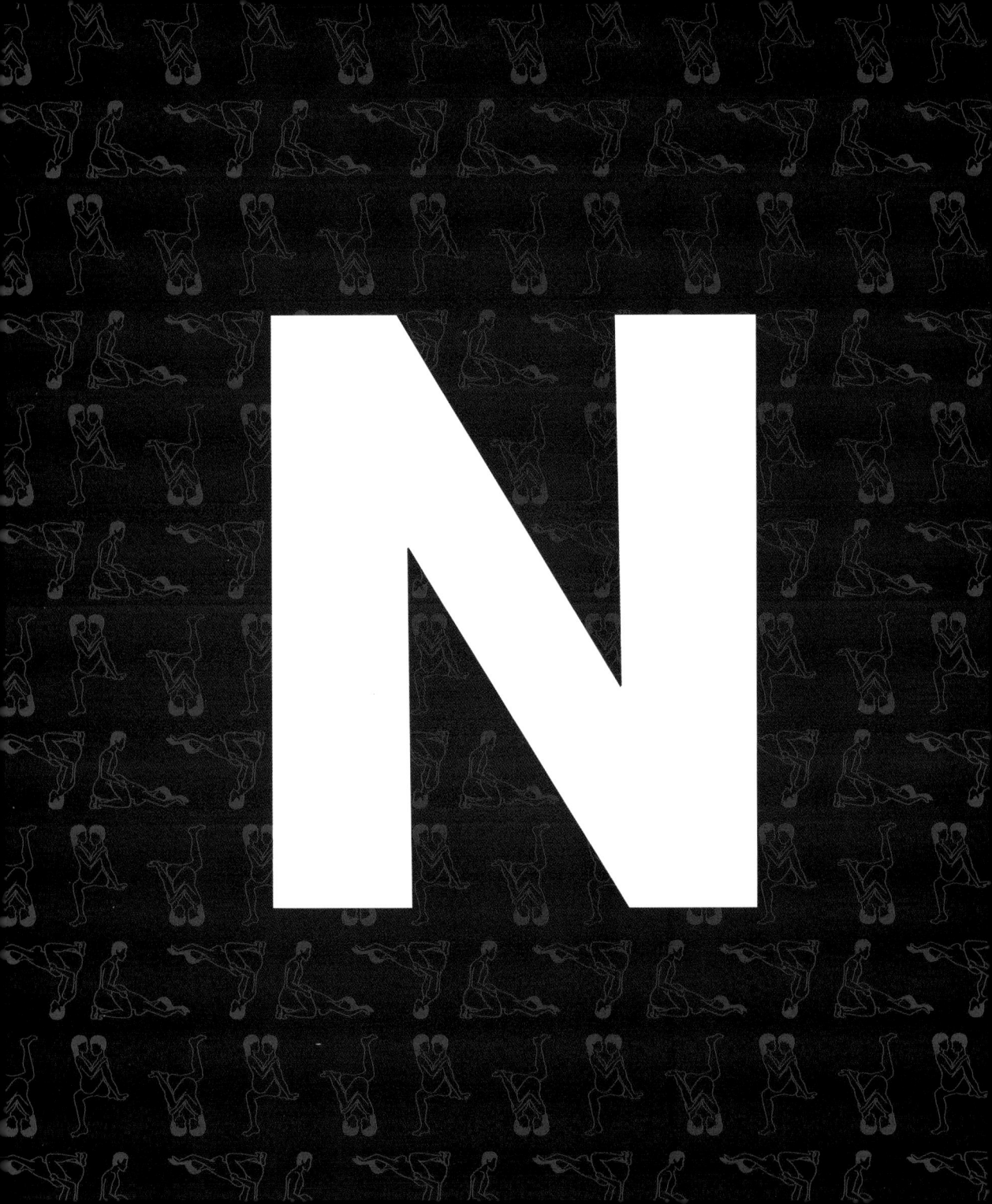

naturist

These days, plenty of young women want to #freethenipple, but naturists (or *nudists*) believe in going further to let it *all* hang out. While a naturist sounds like either someone who studies birds and trees (that would be a *naturalist*!) or someone just looking for an excuse for group sexy time, The Naturist Society (TNS) explains that isn't the case. Actually, for many people, going naked is a much bigger thing and is a "carefully considered way of life."

3 REASONS WHY:

- **It's *really* not about sex.** "Nude is not lewd." Being a naturist is about the freedom nude activities provide rather than bringing sexy back. (You'll probably want to turn to the *orgy* entry, page 137, if this news disappoints you.)

- **It's not about bikini-ready bods.** "Body acceptance is the ideal; nude recreation is the way." The org is clearly chill and inclusive of all shapes and sizes.

- **It's not only about nude sunbathing.** There are so many things you can do nude that you have probably never considered! There are nude backpackers, canoeists, kayakers, scuba divers, and skydivers, as well as nude destinations like nude cruises, resorts, and campgrounds.

RELATED TERMS: *breasts, nipples, orgy, penis*

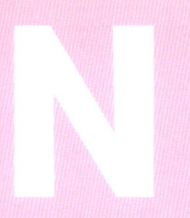

Q: Are my **nipples** normal?

A: First off, to clarify, when we say "nipple," we specifically mean the skin that's nearish the center of your breast, where your breast ducts connect to the surface of your skin. The *areola*, often included in the definition of *nipple*, is the pink- or brown-tinted skin around it. Now back to the question . . .

NIPPLES AND AREOLAE COME IN ALL KINDS OF SIZES.

There's big, small, bumpy, and not-so-bumpy nips, plus a whole bunch of other varieties, none of which are abnormal. It's just how your body developed. So if some jerk ever critiques you for having flat "pepperoni nips," tell him to . . . well, you know what to tell him to do.

The only reason the size or shape of your nipples might be cause for concern is if they become asymmetrical over time. Dr. Sarah P. Cate, a breast surgeon with Mount Sinai Beth Israel, clarified that "a long-term asymmetry is less concerning than an acute one," so if you notice a sudden change in how your nipples match up to one another, you should see a doctor.

If you're deeply concerned about your nipples (for purely aesthetic reasons), there is a surgical procedure to resize them. Dr. Helen Colen, a surgeon with Colen Plastic Surgery in Manhattan, says it involves either removing or adding tissue to the nipple to deflate or puff it up a bit. To make the areola smaller, Dr. Colen explains, surgeons cut around it and then size it down—"just like you'd resize a dress." A tattoo is usually done to make the areola appear bigger, or patients can get a skin graft that takes skin from the inside of their mouth or their labia (YES, OMG, LABIA), but that's a pretty rare choice.

As far as color, anything that isn't clearly irritated skin is normal. Usually your nipples and areolae are a bit darker than the rest of your skin. Dr. Cate says that during the winter, you might get eczema on your nipples, but if they are cracked or red and clearly irritated, you should see a doctor.

WHAT'S THE DEAL WITH THE BUMPS AND HAIR AROUND THE NIPPLES?

There's a lot going on with your areolae. First, there are those little bumps that almost all women have—not the nipples themselves, obvi, but the little pimple-esque bumps around the nipple. Those are called *areolar glands*. They are not pimples, so do not squeeze or try to pop them. Their function is to make little oily secretions that keep the areola and nipple lubricated and protected, and when the nipple is stimulated, they might raise up like goosebumps. Most women have anywhere between four and twenty-eight of these glands around their nipples and areolae.

While some dudes wish women were naturally hairless, the fact is about 30 percent of us have a few little hairs around our areolae. These hairs are very much normal, and a big moment in most female friend groups is the first time you all openly address your nipple hairs with each other. A truly magical time. But if you're really concerned about what others might think when they catch a glimpse of your hair, then yes, it's okay to pluck it. Just do so after your shower, when your pores are open.

SOME NIPS ARE INVERTED.

About 10 percent of women have nipples that don't stick out but instead lie flat or sort of fall back into the breast. These are called *inverted nipples*, and while they might not be "mainstream," they're certainly not harmful or bad. They're just, like, cool indie-alt nipples that listen to bands you've never heard of.

According to Dr. Colen, inverted nipples are a result of the tissue that connects your nipple to your breast being a bit shorter. Dr. Colen also says that, while women can come to her practice to get their inverted nipples surgically everted, inverted nipples are totally functional. Meaning yes, you can breastfeed with inverted nipples, and yes, you can still get turned on when someone plays with your inverted nipples. Having them surgically altered is just an aesthetic choice.

Some women have two inverted nipples, while others might just have one. As Dr. Colen puts it, no two breasts (or nipples) are the same—even when they're on the same woman. But pay close attention to the state of your nips, because according to Dr. Cate, an inverted nipple can, in some cases, be a sign of breast cancer. "If the nipple has previously stuck out and starts to invert, or sink in, this can be a sign," she says. So, if you've noticed a change like that, it can be more serious and you should get it checked out.

As a matter of fact, you should probably give your boobs a self-exam once a month. There are some things to look for, other than breast lumps, that could be signs of cancer. "Dry, cracking skin with bleeding can be indicative of a breast cancer known as Paget's disease," Dr. Cate says. "In addition, spontaneous nipple discharge that comes from one nipple only can be a sign of breast cancer." Even though the average age of breast cancer diagnosis is sixty-one, younger women can get it, too, so don't write off suspicious nipple activity as your nipples being weird.

To sum up: If your nipples have always been the way they are, they're normal. If they've changed a lot recently, or just one has changed, that's not normal and you should take your nipples to a doctor.

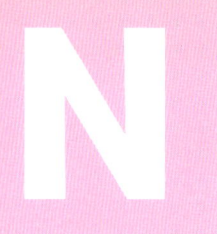

Q: Why do men have **nipples**?

A: Because that's how the male embryo develops. That said, nipples can also enhance a man's orgasm, since they trigger the same zone in a guy's brain as stimulating his penis does, says Barry Komisaruk, PhD. At least, that's the theory. In reality, only 52 percent of dudes have "arousable" nipples, according to a new study. If you're wondering if your man is among that group, try a slow rub with your thumb and forefinger, applying slight pressure before licking all over. If he moans, you've unlocked another one of his hot spots.

✱ **RELATED TERMS:** *breasts, boobgasm, nipple clamps, tune in Tokyo*

nipple clamps

It hurts so good—at least that's what fans of this sex accessory think. These clamps or clips are often sold as "bondage gear" or "sensation play" and vary in intensity from a light pinching feeling (ooh!) to excruciatingly painful (oooouch!). Good Vibrations, the online sex-toy retailer, notes on its website that "nipple clamps squeeze the nipples and . . . when you take them off, the blood that had been squeezed out will return, which can feel really intense." Some clamps are weighted, adjustable, or look like jewelry (with tight little circles surrounding the nipple), and some even have vibrators attached. As with any kind of new bondage gear, however, be sure to take it slowly. And, whether it's you or your partner trying on the nipple clamps, be sure that you are clear on how to safely take them off! (You don't want to have to make an ER run because of a nipple misadventure.)

✱ **RELATED TERMS:** *boobgasm, breasts, BDSM, fetish, kink, nipples, sex toys*

NSFW
This is a commonly used abbreviation for "Not Safe for Work."

nonbinary

Also sometimes called *genderqueer, nonbinary* can be defined as "types of gender identities that cannot be adequately described by male or female and which exist between or outside of those options," according to the Grand Rapids Pride Center (GRPC). GRPC Educational Coordinator Leslie Boker added, "There are many ways to be nonbinary, including genderfluid, bi-gender, and agender."

RELATED TERMS: *androsexuality, asexuality, bisexuality, cisgender, gay, gender, genderqueer, heterosexuality/homosexuality, lesbian, pansexuality, transgender, queer*

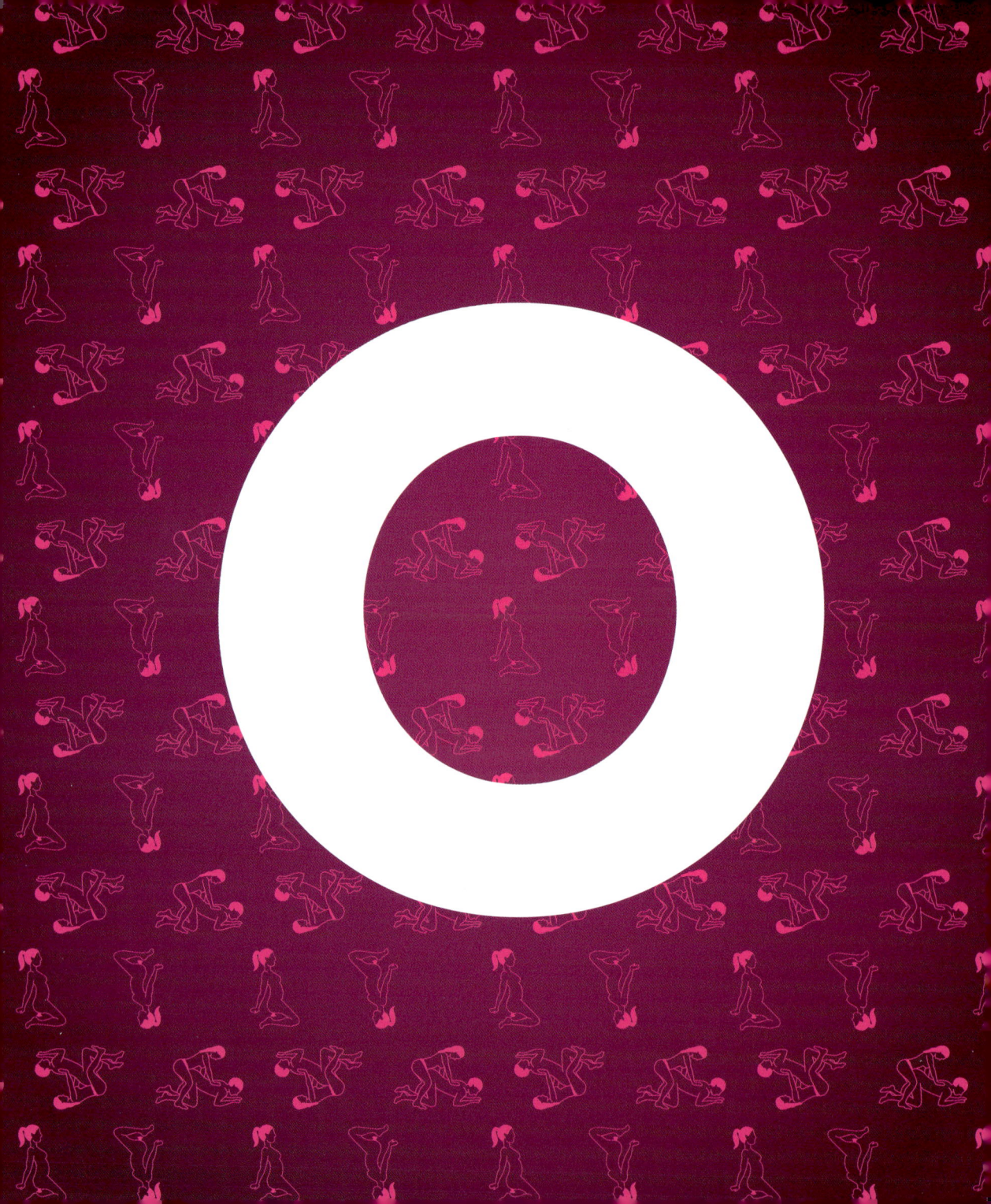

5 things to say and do to get better **oral sex**

The editors of *Cosmo* agree on lots of important stuff—chief among them: Life's too short for bad oral sex. With that in mind, behold these strategic and effective ways of getting exactly the oral you want and deserve.

> FIGURING OUT WHAT YOU LIKE CAN HELP YOU TELL THEM SPECIFICALLY WHAT YOU WANT.

Start off with the right foreplay. Begin by telling them what you want them to do before your clothes are even off—like sexting, but IRL!

Lead with a compliment. Say, "I love it when you do X, can you do that again?" Or say something like "I love when you flick your tongue on my clit." Even if they aren't doing it, maybe they'll start.

Give precise directions. When they have made their way downtown, tell them exactly what you want, using directives like: "Up. To the left. Higher. Lower. Faster. Slower. To the right."

Gently move his head until he's in a spot that feels good. Or move your own hips around until their mouth lines up with a good spot, then say something to make them realize they're in a good spot."

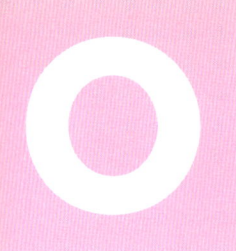

UNFORTUNATELY, ACCORDING TO *COSMO'S* FEMALE ORGASM SURVEY, GOING DOWN DOESN'T EQUAL ORGASM—ONLY 12 PERCENT OF WOMEN COME BY RECEIVING ORAL SEX.

If you pull this off, your partner will think they found this magical spot all on their own. Then use various types of pressure, hair pulling, or dirty talk to keep encouraging them.

Educate yourself on all the different shapes he can make with his tongue. Wide and flat feels differently than sharp and pointy. Figuring out what you like can help you tell them specifically what you want. And if they're already switching things up a lot, like oral roulette or something, wait until they're in a good spot and then affirm that it feels good.

❋ **RELATED TERMS:** *cunnilingus, orgasm*

orgasm

> ON AVERAGE, IT TAKES A WOMAN TWENTY MINUTES TO ORGASM WITH A PARTNER. FOR DUDES? FOUR MINUTES.

There's a lot that goes into getting on your Big O. According to Ian Kerner, PhD, author of *She Comes First*, here's a quick summary of some things that happen on the way to a woman's orgasm, from when you begin to get turned on to the final explosion.

- **During foreplay:** Chemicals and hormones are released, blood flows toward the pelvic area, skin becomes extra sensitive, breasts swell, vulvovaginal glands produce thick fluid, and the clitoris head emerges.

- **Main event:** Blood pressure increases, inner depths of vagina widen and increase at least 2 inches (5 cm) in length, inner labia change color, clitoral head doubles in size, and all the muscular tension that's been building explodes in orgasm—a series of quick, rhythmic contractions. Danish researchers found that the part of the brain that lights up during a heroin rush is also activated during orgasm.

- **Postgame:** According to Kerner, women tend to come down from orgasm slowly—it takes at least 5–10 minutes for women's genitals to return to their non-aroused state. Also, with some stimulation, women are fairly quickly able to go another round.

5 explosive sex positions for more intense **orgasms**

Ready to have deeper, more intense orgasms? You may just need to start mixing some things up to boost your pleasure. Here are advanced sex positions to try.

THE LOW RIDER

If you don't get legendary orgasms from girl-on-top positions, try this: Get on top, but lean back on your hands. It may take a little more balance, but it's worth it because someone (you, him, both) can play with your clit with hand or toy. Rock back and forth and make slow circles with your hips. Oh boy, you shall come hard.

RED LIGHT, GREEN LIGHT

Get in bridge position, lying back with your shoulders on the floor and your hips elevated. He enters, kneeling for superdeep penetration and spot-on friction. (Also, a finger or two curled up inside you instead of a penis is amazing as well.) Use a hand or toy on your clit, and for the most intense orgasm, add a little edging. Just when you're about to lose it, stop for a moment to cool down, then start up again. Repeat 'til you're moaning incoherently.

THE CAT CRAWL

Despite having the least sexy name ever, the Coital Alignment Technique will give you the most intense orgasm you will ever have with a dick inside you. Put a big dollop of lube on your clit and pull back your clitoral hood (speaking of unsexy names) and assume regular missionary position, but have him scooch up just a few inches so his pelvis is resting perfectly on your clit. He does a sexy grind instead of thrusting, and if you put your legs between his for an even tighter fit—crazy intense orgasms for all.

THE HAPPY PUPPY

Get on top, but face toward his feet so you can sort of hump that delicious thigh of his. It is hotter than it sounds, but if his thigh and penis aren't quite doing it for you, add a hand or toy. But . . . if you put a ton of lube on this thigh, it's a lot sexier than you'd guess.

THE THREE-ALARM FIRE

Lie back on a table with something up your butt. Try a butt plug, his finger, or even a dildo if you're an advanced student. He stands between your legs for PnV, then apply your own hand or a small vibrator to your clit. Triple rubbing = magic synergy thing = triple intense orgasm.

→

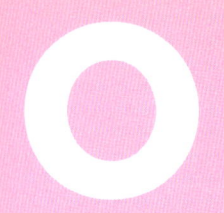

8 surprising reasons you're not **orgasming**

Doctors share the real reasons why you're not getting there.

You're on a medication that is making orgasms nearly impossible. Michael Krychman, MD, executive director of the Southern California Center for Sexual Health, says that medications like SSRIs (selective serotonin reuptake inhibitors; used to treat depression, anxiety, and other conditions) can diminish sex hormones in the body, often leading to having crappy orgasms or no orgasms at all. So if the sex is actually good but the O's just not happening for you, that could be why. Talk to your doctor and see if there's another medication with fewer sexual side effects that you could be taking.

You're only having PNV sex. Dr. Krychman says that a lot of the time, guys think they're incredibly good at sex, but they actually have no idea what they're doing. According to Justin Lehmiller, PhD, author of *The Psychology of Human Sexuality*, only about half of women can orgasm from penetration alone, so it's no wonder you're having problems with the jackhammer method. Try adding in clitoral stimulation via your own hand or a vibrator on your clitoris during sex.

You're not receiving enough foreplay. A lot of women fake orgasms because a lot of men fake foreplay, according to Dr. Krychman. If your guy isn't giving you enough (or any) foreplay, you're never actually getting turned on. So tell him to slow the hell down already and give you time to get there.

You're too stressed out to really enjoy sex. Many women spend a lot of time during sex worried about unintended pregnancy and STIs, as well as whether this guy is good for them or whether he's faithful. According to Raegan McDonald-Mosley, MD, MPH, FACOG, and chief medical officer at Planned Parenthood of Maryland, that makes it really hard for women to let go and be in the moment sexually.

You have no idea what works for you. The vagina has a lot of parts to it, and it's not like we learn a ton about how it all works when we're growing up. Dr. McDonald-Mosley says many women don't even know what feels good to them. She suggests masturbating while stimulating your clitoris and the inside of your vagina at the same time or separately to figure out what you like, and then share with your partner.

You're putting way too much pressure on yourself to have an orgasm quickly. If you're lying there nervous or tired or feeling uncomfortable about how much time has passed, you're creating a vicious cycle of no orgasms. Dr. McDonald-Mosley says that having that pressure to have or give an orgasm just results in everyone being stressed out and not coming. Not ideal. Try not to think about orgasming and just enjoy the sensations instead. You'll come when you least expect it.

You might just need some lube. About 40 percent of women don't produce enough natural lubrication to enjoy sex. Dr. McDonald-Mosley says that even if your body normally gets wet, sometimes the chemistry of condoms, hormones, and emotions can throw that off and leave you dry. Just adding lubricant (ALERT: It's not just for old ladies, it's for every lady) is an easy way to make you feel more comfortable and orgasm-ready.

There's an actual anatomical or physical problem you need to get checked out. True medical problems that affect your ability to orgasm are rare, according to Karen Elizabeth Boyle, MD, FACS, but it is possible to have things like clitoral entrapment, which is when the clitoris literally gets trapped under the clitoral hood skin, making it less sensitive. If you're having significant trouble orgasming, check with your gynecologist to make sure nothing like that is going on. But mostly, Dr. Boyle says it's about finding out what you like via masturbation or toys and then finding a partner who wants to take you there.

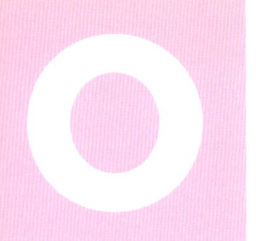

Q: Does a dude's **orgasm** feel as good as a heroin rush?

A: Ever wondered if guys can get addicted to orgasming? It may not seem so far-fetched when you learn some biology. The ventral tegmental area (VTA) plays a crucial role in a wide range of rewarding behaviors and, as study authors noted in the *Journal of Neuroscience*, "because ejaculation introduces sperm into the female reproductive tract, it would be critical for reproduction of the species to favor ejaculation as a most rewarding behavior." So say "no" to drugs and "yes" to . . .

RELATED TERMS: *boobgasm, clitoris, coregasm, edging, ejaculation, fingering, foreplay, fuck, lube, masturbation, PNV, positions, sex toys, sexual intercourse, squirting*

Q: Curious about joining an **orgy?**

A: While classically considered to be group sex with several partners in a party-like scenario, according to Dr. Katherine Frank, author of *Plays Well in Groups: A Journey Through the World of Group Sex*, the word *orgy* insinuates more than just group sex. It hints at something wild and over-the-top. Picture the insane Greek and Roman sex parties that would last for days, where people only paused penetration to eat and sleep.

But modern group sex isn't just pure carnal chaos; there is a lot of prep involved. "The fact is, even at the most spontaneous sex parties, there can be a lot of rules," says Dr. Frank. There are rules about how you ask people, how you disengage, who you can have sex with, what kind of sex you can have."

HERE ARE A FEW THINGS TO KNOW BEFORE YOU GO ORGY HUNTING:

- **The Internet was practically invented for finding info on your local sex groups.** You can explore the BDSM community in particular, which tends to have the hookups when it comes to interesting hookups. Search to find a local dungeon near you (many are reviewed on Yelp!) and see if they have any events or mixers that may be more structured than parties in people's homes.

- **No matter how you find your group sex community, be smart and safe.** Feel free to meet in person with whoever organizes the event in advance to make sure they are trustworthy. Get as much information as you need before committing to an orgy: rules, safe words, condom use, etc. Because an orgy can be a potentially dangerous event if you're not prepared, there are strict rules to keep everyone feeling safe and supported. Getting verbal consent before engaging in any sex acts, using protection, and coming up with safe words are all part of the process.

- **It's not always as easy to get in the sex mix as you think.** A lot of people at sex parties just end up hooking up with whoever they came with. Be patient, and don't feel bad if you aren't instantly the star of the cuddle-puddle.

- **Rejection happens.** Be gracious! Relationship expert Dr. Jess O'Reilly, a veteran of Burning Man's Orgy Dome, says that people at a sex party aren't "going to come up and just dive right in. They'll actually say, 'Can we join you?' or 'Are you guys looking for company?' and they take rejection really surprisingly well."

While play parties and kink scenes can provide entrees into #OrgyLife, you can also start one among friends and people you know simply by asking if they're into the idea. Just be prepared for some awkward conversations and fully acknowledge that your friendships might change after being in a giant, naked heap on top of one another.

RELATED TERMS: *BDSM, fetish, fuck, kink, safe word, sexual intercourse*

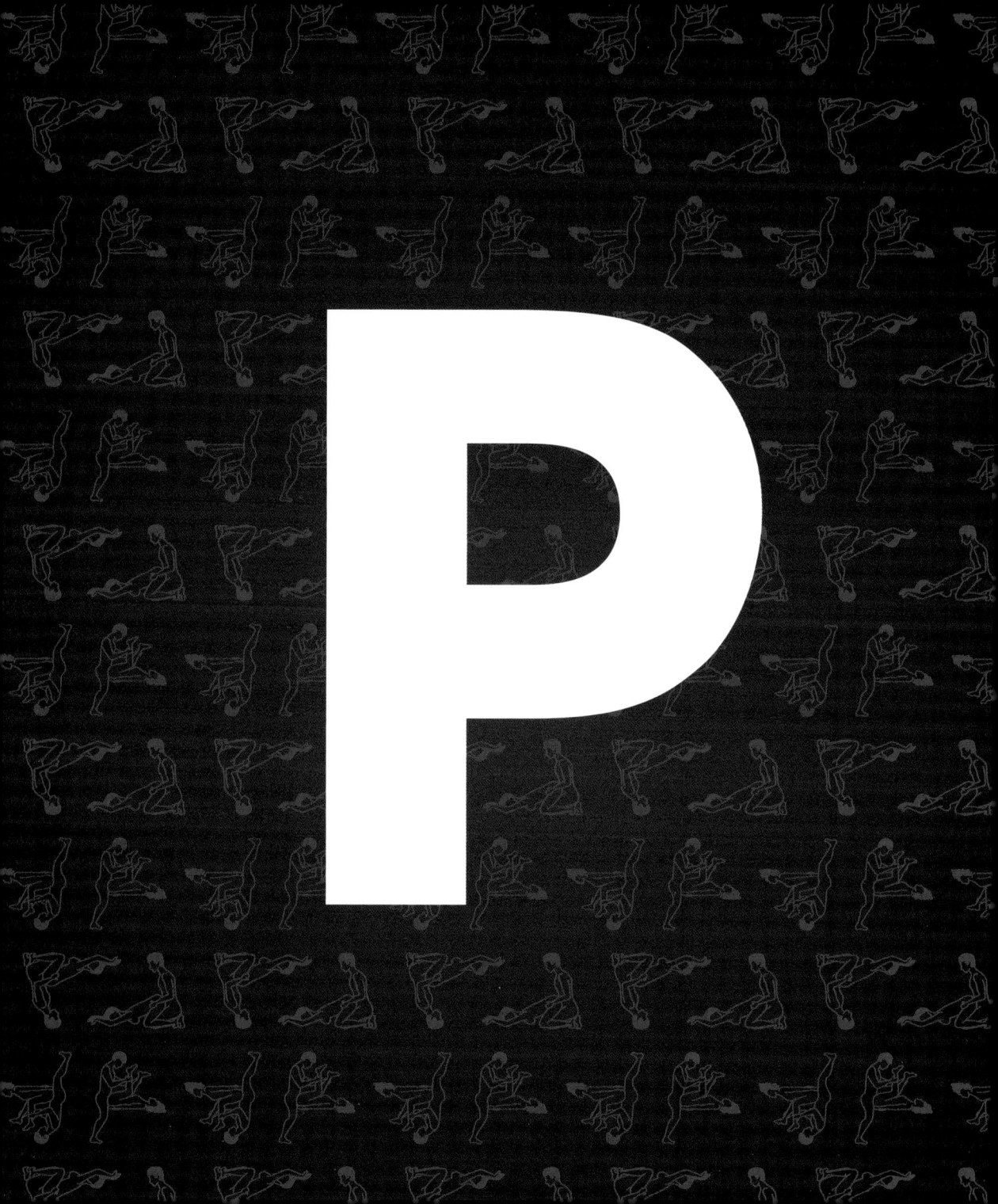

pansexuality

According to the LGBTQ Center at UNC–Chapel Hill, *pansexual* is a term used by some to self-identify that they're attracted to—and may form sexual and romantic relationships with—a person, regardless of that person's gender identity or genitalia. Some use the term *omnisexual* as well.

RELATED TERMS: *androsexuality, asexuality, bisexuality, cisgender, gay, gender, genderqueer, heterosexuality/homosexuality, lesbian, nonbinary, transgender, queer*

P

pearl necklace

Maybe not as classy—and versatile—as the chain of beads you'd wear to high tea, this kind of jewelry is an act during which a man ejaculates onto his partner's neck or chest. The drops of semen are said to look like the individual pearls on a strand of beads. (Ooh, pretty!)

A pearl necklace can be preceded by any sort of sexual act capable of making a man come. However, because of proximity, acts that happen close to the neck or chest area, like breast screwing or blow jobs, often end in a pearl necklace. Plus, we think it's a great alternative to a facial if you're not ready for that level of

If you're in charge of the penis—aka, if you are the one giving a blow job or hand job—just make sure you aim it onto your neck and chest at the appropriate moment. You can do this by requesting your partner tell you when he's about to come. If you're letting him make that game-time decision, make sure you've communicated your desire about where that ejaculate lands, so you don't end up with it six inches higher than you were hoping.

✱ **RELATED TERMS:**
cum, ejaculation, facial, oral sex,

> PEGGING IS ABOUT MORE THAN JUST TOYS: IT INVOLVES PSYCHOLOGICAL AROUSAL, AS WELL AS PHYSICAL.

pegging

Pegging has something to do with stabilizing a country's currency, according to Investopedia. This *isn't* that.

In sexual terms, pegging is when a woman performs anal intercourse on a man with the help of a strap-on dildo. A woman can also peg another woman. The term was coined fifteen years ago when sex columnist Dan Savage ran a contest back in 2001 asking readers to vote on a name for the act. (The losers were *bobbing* and *punting*.) "There are lots of stereotypes and myths about pegging, the most common being that if you like it, you must be gay," says Tristan Taormino, a sex educator and author of eight books, including *The Ultimate Guide to Anal Sex for Women*. "You can just really love anal pleasure, and it won't change your sexual orientation." Taormino notes that prostate stimulation, which is what pegging accomplishes in men, is a "gateway to amazing orgasms" for dudes.

Once both people decide they are game, the first step is shopping for the right toy. You want to find a harness and strap-on that are comfortable for the pegger to wear and, of course, comfortable for the person being pegged. "I always say 'he picks the dick,'" Taormino says.

It's important for the partner who's being penetrated to take the lead and control the pace. Communication and patience are key, as is lots of lube. Seriously, use lots. Doggy style is obviously an easy position to peg in, but feel free to mix it up. There are as many fun pegging positions as there are colors of the rainbow. One favorite is reverse cowboy, which is where a dude sits on your lap, facing away from you as you take him from behind. Whatever position you land on, flipping the script on traditional gender roles can be a fun way to spice it up.

The variations mainly depend on the type of dildo you choose. There are large ones, small ones, realistic-looking ones, and vibrating ones. But pegging is about more than just toys: It involves psychological arousal, as well as physical. "It's really exciting for women to experience this new kind of sex and to be the penetrator," Taormino says. "Likewise, it's exciting for men to experience a whole new kind of pleasure of being penetrated, which can change the sexual game."

✱ RELATED TERMS: *anal, anal play, dildo, lube, sex toys*

penis

10 FACTS TO KNOW

Peen, wang, dick, cock, willy, schlong, or dong: No matter what you like to call it, there are as many nicknames for his D as there are myths about how it actually works. We spoke with Benjamin Brucker, MD, assistant professor of urology at NYU Langone Medical Center, to lay down some phallic knowledge. Here's what he shared.

There's really no difference between circumcised and uncircumcised penises.
The only discernable difference between circumcised and uncircumcised penises is the likelihood of developing penile cancer (it's rare in general, but uncircumcised men are at a higher risk). Uncircumcised men are also slightly more likely to transmit HPV and HIV to partners if they don't use a condom. Those bummers aside, most of the assumptions people have about circumcision affecting penis size and sexual prowess are myths. "Being uncircumcised really should not affect the size of the penis; it's just the appearance," says Dr. Brucker. The foreskin probably pulls back a bit during vaginal penetration, so I don't know if there's anything they would necessarily notice." It's really just personal preference: Do you prefer your convertibles with the hood up or down?

Penises can break.
"It's called a penile fracture. You would think of a bone fracturing because that's what most fractures are described as, but the fracture in the penis comes from the fibrous tissue of the penis essentially developing a rip or a tear in it," says Dr. Brucker. Because we all know the penis is not a bone or a muscle, but an

organ, right? Right! "Sometimes in medical textbooks, they'll call [a broken penis] an *eggplant deformity* or an *eggplant* because it will actually turn purple, bruised, and take on that shape of an eggplant."

They're more resilient than you think.
It might be easy to do some damage to a penis with an accidental bite or an overzealous grip, but don't worry about doing any permanent damage. Going limp is the penis's natural reaction if a guy is in any kind of pain. "The good news about the penis is that it has a lot of blood flow in most men, so it heals well and allows your immune system to work," says Dr. Brucker. "But just like any other part of your body, it needs to be treated appropriately and you don't want to be too aggressive."

Men can get yeast infections and UTIs, too.
Typically, you're not going to pass yeast infections or urinary tract infections (UTIs) to your partner, although it can happen. "A female urethra is usually about four centimeters, and the man's urethra is longer. Some guys can get topical yeast infections; it's usually just a skin irritation. When a man gets a urinary tract infection, there's usually a problem going on, like an enlarged prostate," explains Dr. Brucker.

Erectile dysfunction is usually indicative of other health issues.
Stress, drugs (prescription or otherwise), alcohol, age, and obesity can all cause ED. It can even be a sign of diabetes or heart disease. "Once you start to see erectile dysfunction, the first thing you should evaluate is his overall health," says Dr. Brucker.

No one actually knows the average penis size.
There's no standard tool for measuring a penis and no easy way of doing so. Some studies stretch the penis out by tying a weight to it (*oy*); others measure from the base of the prepubic area as opposed to the base of the penis. And penises are always changing size. "A large portion of the penis is actually inside of the body and then there's also the distinction between when you're measuring the penis of a man who has a little bit of weight in the pubic hair area or not. You can have a guy with the actual same penis length and he's superskinny—the portion of the penis measured may appear to be longer versus a guy with a little weight on him."

P

The clitoris is basically a tiny penis.
"In embryologic development, the penis and the clitoris actually evolve from the same tissue. So the clitoris can technically become erect," explains Dr. Brucker. Basically, everyone starts with vaginal lips in the womb, and if the Y chromosome is present, things start flipping around like a genital Transformer. "The ovaries, or the gonads, descend and become the testicles, the labia fuse and become the scrotum, and then the clitoris enlarges and becomes the penis." Wild.

There's really no scientific basis for the idea of a guy being a "grower, not a shower."
Every penis is different. "You can have a man with a small penis who gets erections and is large, or a man with a small penis who gets erect and it doesn't grow more. Or you can have a man with a large penis who gets erect but it doesn't grow any more. Or you can have a man with a large penis who gets erect and it grows more," says Dr. Brucker. Judge not the penis that neither grows nor shows.

The average guy can last about five minutes.
"Men think they're supposed to be able to last an hour and a half or two hours, but the reality is most women would say at that point, sex becomes uncomfortable. Most of the time sex lasts minutes, not hours," says Dr. Brucker.

Men can't always get continual erections, because their penises basically just ran a marathon.
Every penis is different. Some can do back-to-back sex sessions, and others need to take a break and rehydrate. It's what's known as a *refractory period*. "The refractory period is just part of normal physiology. Different parts of your nervous system are working for erections and ejaculation, and it's hard or your body to switch back and forth quickly. The refractory time varies a lot based on age and other issues," says Dr. Brucker. Don't be disappointed if the penis needs a break every once in a while. It's just extra time for him to go down on you or try something new.

RELATED TERMS: *balls, circumcision, genitalia, M-zone, pubic hair, uncircumcised*

piercings

PNV
A commonly used abbreviation for sex that involves inserting a penis in a vagina.

Curious about getting your privates pierced? Is your dude interested in accessorizing his junk? According to tattoo and piercing site Painful Pleasures, here are the basics on common genital piercings to get you thinking (or shrieking):

- **Apadravya:** goes through the head of the penis from top to bottom

- **Ampallang:** goes through the head of the penis from side to side

- **Christina or Venus:** a surface piercing done vertically on the pubic mound above the clitoral hood

- **Clitoral:** The clitoris can be pierced, but it's rarely done because the outcome can often be extreme: (a) nerves in the clitoris may be damaged, desensitizing a woman temporarily or permanently, or (b) it can cause such constant overstimulation that it could drive a woman to distraction.

- **Frenum:** Side-to-side surface piercings placed along the underside of the penis shaft; frenum piercings can be stimulating for partners during intercourse.

- **Guiche:** These are perineum surface piercings (i.e., piercings of the area between the testicles and anus). The perineum is an erogenous zone for many men, so this piercing has the potential to be more physically stimulating than others.

- **Hafada/scrotum:** These are surface piercings placed anywhere on the scrotum. They're often done as a "ladder," with several piercings done in a column. Some men attach a small weight to the piercing to pull the scrotal sack down during sex, which can prolong orgasm.

- **Inner and outer labia:** An outer labia piercing goes through one of the outer vaginal lips, and an inner labia piercing goes through one of the inner lips. Some women will get just one side pierced, but most get labia piercings in pairs. Others work toward two matching rows of 3–5 rings or tunnels.

- **Prince Albert piercing:** goes through the underside of the head of the penis, into the urethra, and out through the urethral opening

- **Reverse Prince Albert piercings:** Some men prefer to have their PA piercings go through the urethra from the top of the penis head instead of the underside, either for their partner's benefit or aesthetics.

RELATED TERMS:
balls, fourchette, genitalia, penis, vagina, VCH

polyamory

"The more the merrier" is not just a chill sign-off to your party invite. It's also a sex-and-love philosophy. Some even consider it to be a sexual orientation. Polyamory is the practice of having multiple romantic partners, with the basic idea being: Why limit yourself to just one person at a time when there are so many fabulous people you could love/bone?

But if you want a more textbook definition, according to Elisabeth Sheff, PhD, author of *The Polyamorists Next Door: Inside Multiple-Partner Relationships and Families*, polyamory is "a form of consensual nonmonogamy that emphasizes emotional connection among multiple partners."

There are infinite ways to design a poly relationship, but a common element is the existence of a *primary partner*. The Polyamory Society website defines the primary relationship as "the closest relationship type, the person(s) given the most time, energy, and priority in a person's life." It's basically a person's main squeeze. After that is the *secondary partner*, which, as the title suggests, means they get less time, attention, and commitment than the primary partner. And it goes down the line from there.

Polyamory can take on a multitude of forms. Sometimes, it's two heterosexual couples who switch off spouses without any same-sex sexual interaction; sometimes it's a group of several people where every member is intimate with one another; and sometimes it's a pair of people with one shared secondary partner.

The term *polyfidelity* refers to a group of more than two people who are all connected to each other emotionally or sexually, but who have a closed relationship otherwise. That means that if four people are in a polyfidelity relationship, they are allowed

10 STEPS TO INSURE SUCCESSFUL

Define your terms.

Be honest with yourself and your partners.

State your boundaries, and make rules and agreements.

Start slow and be gentle with yourself—it takes time and work.

Safe sex is a must, obvi.

to sleep with one another but not with anyone else outside their foursome. Then there's *polyaffectivity*, which "emphasizes the emotional connection among people who are not lovers but share a lover in common," says Sheff, who originated the term. Sheff describes the most common polyaffective relationship dynamic as "a woman with two male partners who are emotionally close but not lovers."

If you're interested in trying a polyamorous relationship, first check out these tips from Barbara Carrellas, sex coach and educator and author of *Urban Tantra*.

❋ **RELATED TERMS:** *consensual nonmonogamy, orgy*

Q: What's the difference between an open relationship and a **poly** relationship?

A: The main diff, according to Laurie Ellington, founder of the polyamorous relationship website Poly Coach, is that in an open relationship, there is always a primary partnership. With polyamory, there doesn't have to be. In a poly relationship between three people (known as a *triad*), everyone could love one another equally. In an open relationship, there is a committed couple at the center.

POLYAMOROUS RELATIONSHIPS

Push yourself out of your comfort zone and welcome personal growth.

State your needs clearly.

Keep things clear and transparent.

Prioritize and keep in mind what is best for everyone involved.

You can always renegotiate, redefine, or change things up.

Q: What is a **pompoir** and how is it different from kegels?

A: The act of using the vaginal muscles in different ways to stimulate the penis during intercourse is called *pompoir* (which some pronounce *pompwahr*). Basically, it's Pilates for your vagina. It's historically an act meant to give pleasure to a male partner, although strengthening the vaginal walls can help with incontinence and bladder health as well (score!).

According to Denise Da Costa, a pompoir expert and the author of *Pompoir: The Ultimate Guide to Pelvic Floor Fitness*, "it improves the sexual experience for both the woman and her partner." In her book, Da Costa describes several different movements a woman can learn to do with the vaginal wall muscles that involve squeezing, contracting, pushing, pulling, and a combination of these. Pompoir is often described as "milking" the penis. The act has origins in ancient India and has also been referenced in Arabic culture. According to Da Costa, pompoir originated in the ancient tradition of Hindu dancers, called *devadasis*. "It is mostly known in Far Eastern cultures, but it does not appear to have achieved what we would consider mainstream acceptance," she explains.

But even though pompoir seems similar to Kegel exercises, Da Costa explains that it's very different. Kegel exercises focus primarily on squeezing, whereas a pompoir focuses on four different motions—

> **"THE DIFFERENT MOTIONS MAKE A MORE COMPLETE WORKOUT AND ALLOW THE WOMAN TO BETTER CONTROL THE INTIMACY BETWEEN HER AND HER PARTNER.**

squeeze, contract, push, and pull. "The different motions make a more complete workout and allow the woman to better control the intimacy between her and her partner."

One pompoir exercise you can try at home is something that Da Costa calls twisting. "The easiest way to explain this is if you hold a pen between your thumb and pointer finger. You then move them in opposite directions, twisting the pen. You do the same concept with your vaginal muscles on your partner's genitals." At worst, you're doing it wrong, but you still get to have sex! Sounds worth it.

There are other exercises that include an elaborate program using toys, such as a straight vibrating rod, Ben Wa balls, and other items that you insert into the vagina and manipulate internally. "*Manipulate* in this context means to move the male genitalia with the vaginal muscles to control the experience for the male partner," Da Costa explains. "For example, by contracting the vaginal muscles, it is like a woman is caressing the male genitalia. If the woman squeezes, it is more like a kissing sensation. So the woman is manipulating the experiences felt by her partner." Da Costa recommends practicing pompoir for an hour a day to see results.

★ **RELATED TERMS:**
Kegel, sex toys, vagina

P

Crazy hot positions

You've probably got your missionary and your cowgirl down cold, but if you're feeling a little bored in the bedroom, you've come to the right place. We at *Cosmo* are experts—okay, some might even say obsessed—with sex positions. Here are a few variations on everything from solo action to light S&M.

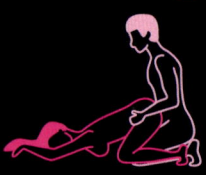

IF YOU'RE CURIOUS ABOUT A LITTLE SEXY DISCIPLINE …

Always wanted to try out spanking but never really knew how to ease into it? Try this entry-level posish for optimal control. Get on your hands and knees on a bed or couch with him behind you. Make sure

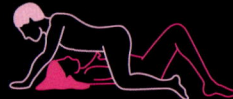

IF YOUR BREASTS NEED SOME LOVIN' …

While on your back or seated with your back up (and with copious amounts of lube, because chafing is REAL), have your dude rub himself in between your breasts while you touch yourself—and watch him go. It's like seeing a Broadway show in a small theatre—every seat has a good view! Another option is to have your guy sit on a chair

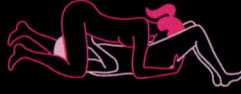

IF YOU LIKE TO MULTITASK IN BED …

Consider this a sexier version of the classic 69. Have your dude lie on his back while you straddle him and give him an upside-down beej. Stick your booty up and out so he can use your favorite toy or his fingers to bring you to completion, all

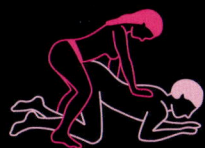

IF YOU'RE INTO PEGGING …
For this, you need to strap on a dildo and use plenty of lube. He's bent over—ass-up on the bed—in a submissive position, and it's easy to give him a firm spanking if he's been a bad boy. Plus, he can control the speed at which he takes your strap-on and keep a hand free to play with himself.

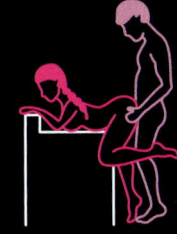

IF YOU'RE IN A HURRY …
Strip down naked and bend over a couch/side of the bed/stool/laundry hamper/whatever, and flash your ass at your dude. Be sure to brace yourself as he takes you from behind, and don't forget to look behind you every so often to admire the curve of your own back.

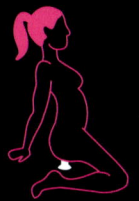

IF YOU'RE READY FOR A SOLO WORKOUT …
Pop a squat on a suction-cup dildo affixed to the surface of your choice and go to town. Even if you don't orgasm from penetration, that doesn't mean it can't still feel AMAZING. Plus, for the normally shy, this lets you act out all your wild sex fantasies without an audience—for now.

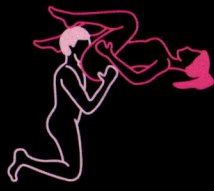

IF HE NEEDS TO UP HIS ORAL GAME …
Lay on the side of your bed on your back with one leg up and one leg down. Have your guy go to town on you while kneeling against the bed. This position leaves you wide open and frees up your dude's neck muscles from getting a cramp so he can keep doing that thing you like even longer.

P

10 most popular **positions**

According to a survey of women in the US and UK, conducted by UK online doctor service Zava, the top-ten most-popular positions, including some oral options, are:

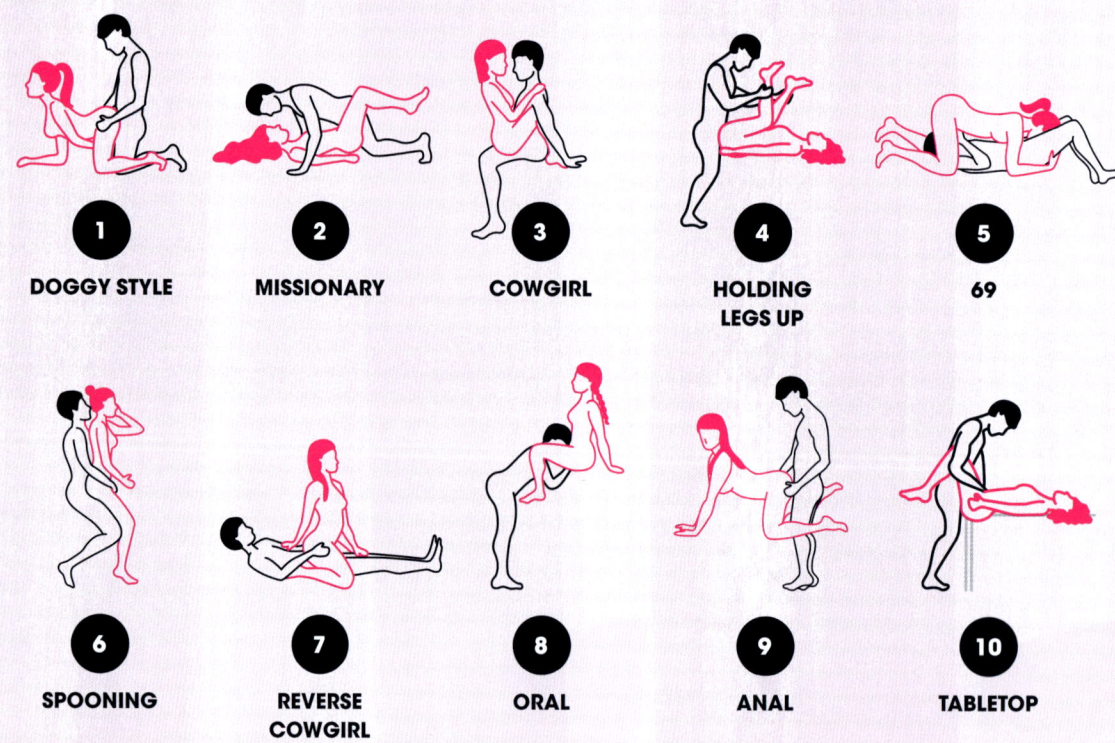

1. DOGGY STYLE
2. MISSIONARY
3. COWGIRL
4. HOLDING LEGS UP
5. 69
6. SPOONING
7. REVERSE COWGIRL
8. ORAL
9. ANAL
10. TABLETOP

✱ **RELATED TERMS:** *anal, anal play, doggy style, fuck, kama sutra, missionary, oral sex, orgasm, quickie, rough sex, sexual intercourse, shower sex, tantric sex*

precum

Also known as *pre-ejaculate*, this clear, colorless fluid seeps from a man's penis when sexually aroused. Similar in composition to semen, pre-cum lacks sperm. But can it get you pregnant? That's up for debate as the science is inconclusive, so best to play it safe and use a condom all throughout intercourse. As for STI transmission, HIV, gonorrhea, chlamydia, and Hepatitis B can be spread via pre-ejaculate.

★ **RELATED TERMS:** *cum*, *STI*

5 pressing **pubic hair** questions, answered

For something that occupies such a tiny plot on the body, there's a lot of talk about pubic hair. And a lot of confusion! To clarify, we asked two doctors to weigh in on what you need to know.

Why do people have pubic hair? While there are theories as to why pubes exist, the most common one is that they likely developed to "protect the genitals against friction during sexual intercourse," according to Leah Millheiser, MD, an OB/GYN and director of the Female Sexual Medicine Program at Stanford University. Another popular theory is that the arrival of pubic hair signaled to potential mates that a partner was able to reproduce. A third theory—and perhaps an argument against going bare—is that pubes act as a "scent trap" for smells in the genital area that could help attract a sexual partner.

What's the best way to shave? The skin in your pubic area is extra sensitive, and the hair is a bit coarser than other body hair. The combination of those two facts can mean that shaving there gets a bit dicey. Joshua Zeichner, MD, a dermatologist in New York City, advises that the best time to shave your pubic hair is in the shower, but not right after you get in—wait a while. "The humidity and warmth of the water helps hydrate and soften both the skin and the hair, allowing shaving to be an easier process," Dr. Zeichner says. He also recommends shaving with the direction of the hair. Shaving against the grain may give a closer shave but it increases the risk of ingrown hairs and razor bumps. "Take short, single strokes, and rinse off the razor every one to two shaves," Dr. Zeichner says. Rinsing the razor is an important step, as a clogged razor is more likely to leave the ends of your pubic hair ragged, and ragged ends are more likely to become irritated.

Both Dr. Zeichner and Dr. Millheiser say it's important to have a razor you use only for your pubes, and it needs to be sharp to remove the thicker pubic hair. Ideally, use one that's shaped to more nimbly navigate the vulva, such as a "bikini razor." Equally important is how you take care of the skin afterward. "Razor burn is essentially inflammation of the skin from shaving," Dr. Zeichner says, so moisturizing after is helpful.

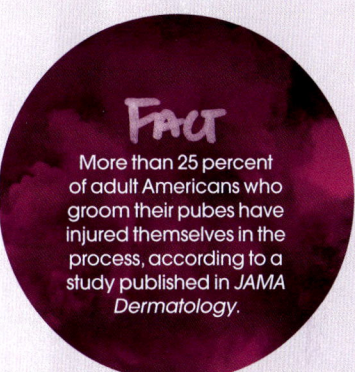

FACT
More than 25 percent of adult Americans who groom their pubes have injured themselves in the process, according to a study published in *JAMA Dermatology*.

What's the deal with ingrown hairs? Ingrown hairs happen when the free edge of a hair gets trapped back into the skin, says Dr. Zeichner. The risk is higher if the skin is inflamed or if you're using a dull razor, which leaves a jagged edge on the hair that's more likely to grow back into the skin. To avoid ingrown hairs, Dr. Zeichner suggested shaving in the direction the hair grows and taking care of skin after shaving with a good moisturizer.

Is it healthy to be bare, or do you need pubic hair? Dr. Millheiser says it's perfectly okay to be bare, but shaving or waxing may put women in particular at risk for bacterial infections or STIs, due to small tears in the skin caused by these procedures that allow for easier transmission of viruses and bacteria.

How often do most women wax or shave their pubic hair? This number widely varies and largely depends on personal preference, rate of growth, and age. A Cosmopolitan.com survey found that women are more likely than men to groom pubic hair in some capacity at least once a week. And women also tend to spend more on said grooming—55 percent of women said they spend $1 to $20 a month on pube-grooming, while 67 percent of men said they spend zilch.

★ **RELATED TERMS:** *anal bleaching, hair removal, labia*

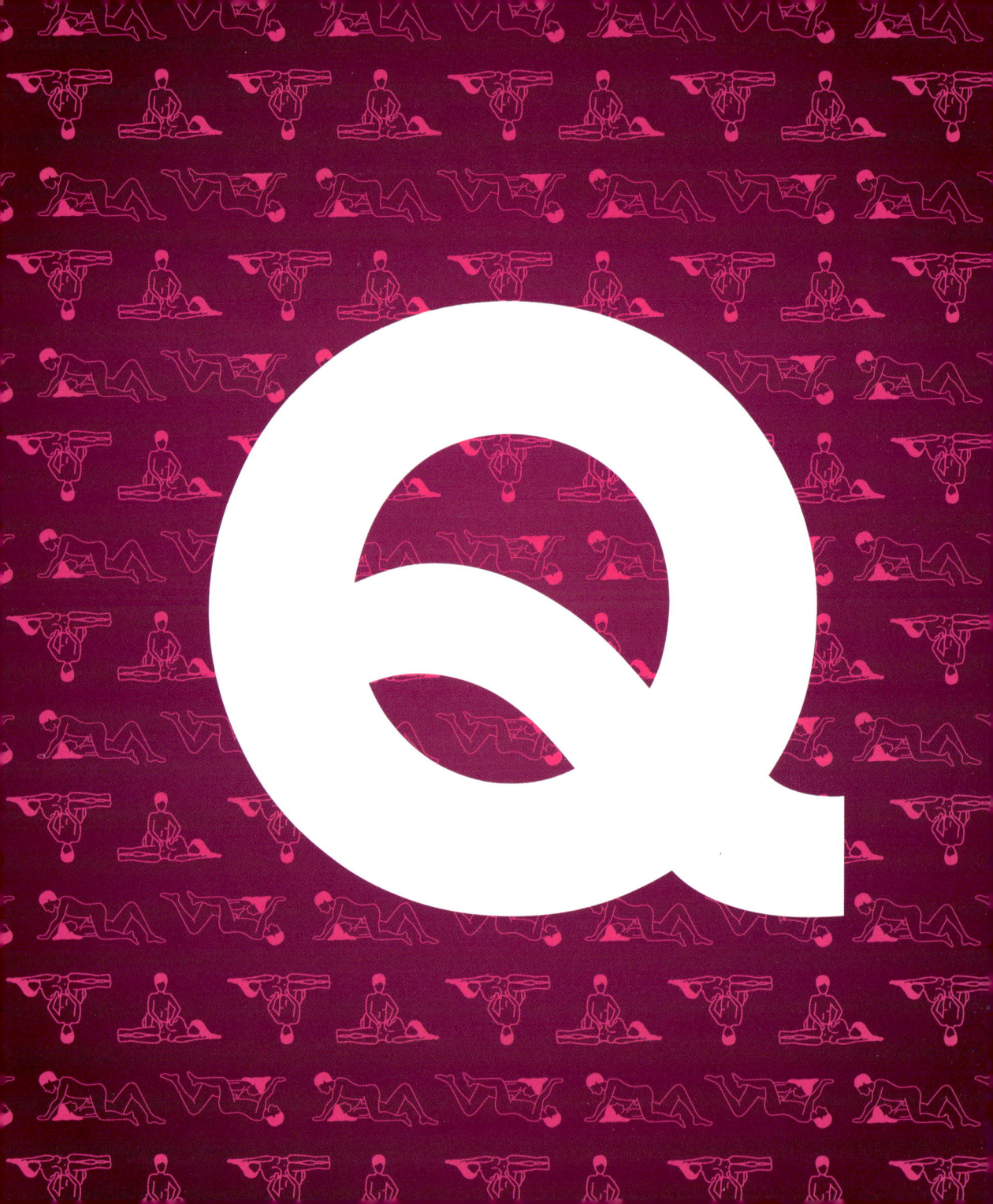

9 things to know about **queefing**

Or make that 10 if you've never heard of it. Queefing happens when air gets trapped in your vagina—and it's a totally natural bodily function.

But somehow, no matter how often you remind yourself that it's natural, it's still difficult not to blush a little when it happens. Here, San Jose–based board-certified OB/GYN Sheila Loanzon, DO, answers everything you've ever wanted to know about queefing and explains why you should never be ashamed.

It's not a fart. Dr. Loanzon says a queef is just the passage of air through the vaginal canal. A queef happens when air pushed into the vagina from something like sexual penetration (be it from a toy or a penis) needs to be released.

You hear vibrations. "The sound comes from the vibrations of the labia majora, which includes the vulva and vaginal lips." Dr. Loanzon explains. "It's similar to the sound of *flatus*, colloquially known as farting, or gas exiting from the rectum, which occurs when the butt cheeks flap together."

You can't hold in queefs like farts. "The anal sphincter is much tighter and better toned than the vaginal tissue and therefore can be controlled," Dr. Loanzon says. "It can contain passage of gas from the gastrointestinal tract, whereas you can't control your vaginal muscles as readily."

Certain positions will put you more at risk than others. Dr. Loanzon says moves like doggy style, in which your partner pushes more air into your vaginal canal, can make you more prone to queefing than others. You can also be more likely to queef if you rotate positions too quickly.

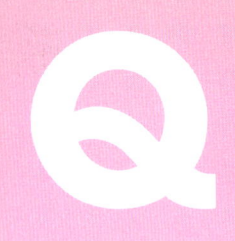

5 Your medical history may also make you more likely to queef. Dr. Loanzon says women who have given birth to larger babies may have larger vaginal canals, which can accommodate more air.

6 There's really nothing you can do about queefing. "If you try to contract the vaginal canal to prevent air from coming in, it can cause sex to be more painful," Dr. Loanzon explains. "If anything, you could try to manage it by slowing down the speed of penetration and using less depth—not having sex hard and fast, jackhammer-style—but it's probably not that realistic in the heat of the moment."

7 Using a lot of lube can mean delayed queefs. Dr. Loanzon says if air bubbles get trapped inside lube, a queef can come out during sex or when urinating afterward.

8 You can queef from doing nonsexual things, like jumping jacks, coughing, or even wearing underwear. Yep! Dr. Loanzon says anything that can introduce air into the vagina, like jumping jacks, trampolining, coughing, and sneezing, can also lead to queefing. "Some people also notice that when they're wearing a thong, the labia gets trapped, and air can get in that way, too. That's another reason why you shouldn't be embarrassed, because it usually happens when you're either having sex, exercising, or wearing clothes, which means you're taking care of yourself in some way."

9 The word *queef* is not a medical term. Dr. Loanzon says doctors normally just refer to it as the "passage of air through the vaginal canal."

✸ **RELATED TERMS:** *fuck, labia, lube, sexual intercourse, vagina*

queening

All women deserve to rule their bedrooms, and the good news is that this oral sex move can help you do just that. At *Cosmo*, we call it the "All Hail The Queen" position, otherwise known as a little old-fashioned face-sitting.

The best thing about sitting on someone's face is you can get both an orgasm and a thigh workout! It's a twofer! Face-sitting, just to be clear, is when a woman dangles her genitals over her partner's mouth for some intense oral sex.

Face-sitting is particularly big in the BDSM community, which is where it earned the nickname *queening*, as in a queen sitting on her throne. There are worse ways to spend a Sunday. Here's how to do it:

If you are the queen, you can kneel over your "subject," who will be lying down on their back. Straddle their face with your legs and use your thigh muscles to hover your genitals right over their mouth. You don't want to put your full weight on their face or you could restrict their breathing, which is dangerous. As far as which direction to face, it's entirely up to you; it doesn't make a lick of difference.

Once you are in position, your partner should do whatever they normally do when giving cunnilingus. This includes, but is not limited to, sucking, kissing, and flicking your clit with their tongue. Feel free to take advantage of this empowering posish to tell your partner what you want. After all, you are the queen.

RELATED TERMS:
BDSM, clit, cunnilingus, oral sex

Q

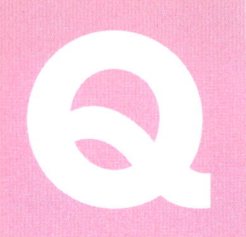

queer

According to the LGBTQ Center at the University of North Carolina at Chapel Hill, *queer* is a term with varied meanings. It has been used as derogatory slang for the LGBTQ community, but "in the early 1990s, many individuals and organizations began to reclaim this term. Some people use it as an all-inclusive or umbrella term to refer to all people who identify as LGBTIQA+—often meant to be an abbreviation for lesbian, gay, bisexual, transgender, intersex, queer (or questioning), ally (or asexual). [The plus is often added to include individuals who don't feel represented by the rest of the letters.] This usage is not accepted by the entire community. [The term is] often used by people who wish to challenge norms of sexuality and/or gender expression as well as to defy identities and labeling of persons."

RELATED TERMS: *androsexuality, asexuality, bisexuality, cisgender, gay, gender, genderqueer, heterosexuality/homosexuality, lesbian, nonbinary, pansexuality, transgender*

quickie

If tantric sex is a triathlon, a quickie is the 50-meter dash. Like the name insinuates, a *quickie* is speedy, rushed sex without all the bells and whistles of foreplay before or cuddling afterward. It's basically the fast food of fucking. Good once in a while, but might leave you feeling gross if you have it all the time. Carol Queen, staff sexologist at online sex-toy store Good Vibrations, points out, though, that the term *quickie* is relative based on how long sex normally lasts for you.

Superspeedy sex is often associated with a situation in which a couple is so horny that they have to bone down ASAP because they can't wait another second. "The initial arousal of both people can help to make it a satisfying sexual encounter even though it doesn't last very long or give a lot of time for build-up of arousal," Queen says.

A few situations can heighten the excitement of a quickie, says Queen. For example, if you're at a party and run into the bathroom for a quickie, the sneaky aspect of it can be really hot.

Another element that can heat things up is the prospect of exhibitionism, such as having sex at the gym or in an empty changing room. For some people, this may be terrifying, and for others, the risk of getting caught makes it that much more thrilling. Just remember, sex in even semipublic places can be illegal, so proceed with caution—especially if you're somewhere with cameras potentially recording your every move and moan.

🌟 **RELATED TERMS:**
fuck, sexual intercourse

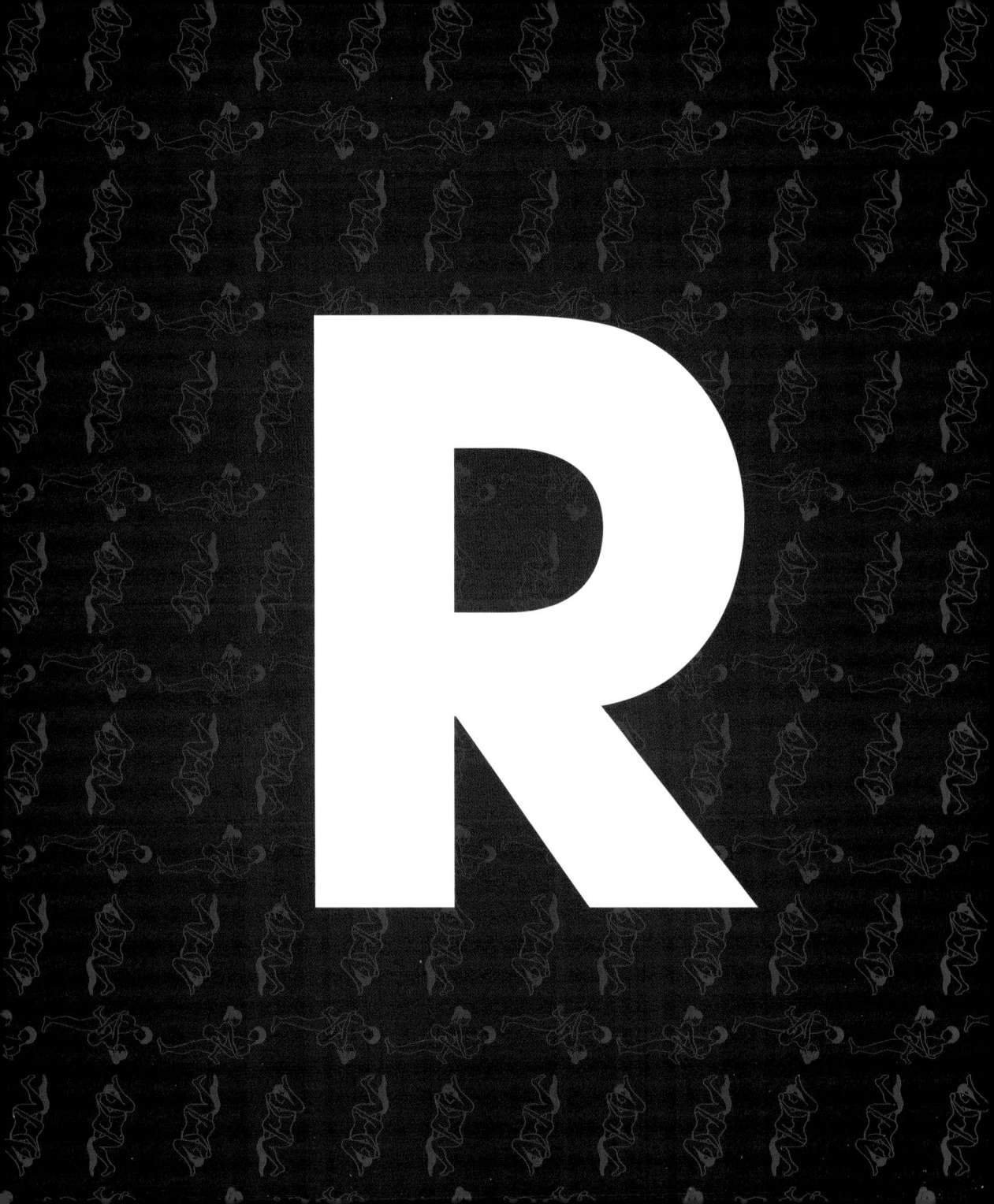

> IT'S LIKE NAP TIME FOR A DUDE'S D.

Q: What is a **refractory** period?

A: Post-orgasm, most men aren't able to get an erection again for a while. In general, the younger the guy, the shorter the period, although there are some who can go again virtually right away and others who need an entire day.

If you want round two ASAP, use your mouth and hands on his other hot spots to recharge his arousal. "Continue kissing and caressing his shoulders, chest, and back," says sexologist Emily Morse, host of the podcast *Sex with Emily*. "His member might need a break, but his brain will be receptive, and eventually, you'll be able to tell when he's coming back online." Boing! Or while you wait, have him pleasure you instead.

✱ **RELATED TERMS:** *ejaculation, erection, orgasm, penis*

R

4 major perks to **reverse cowgirl**

As you probably already know very well, the cowgirl sex position involves having your guy lie on his back with you facing forward, straddling him. The reverse cowgirl is exactly what it sounds like—with you facing in the other direction. But there are ways to maximize the hell out of reverse cowgirl.

You're in control, so mix things up and do whatever feels best.

You can vary the speed and depth of penetration. Or play with your movements by gyrating back and forth or in circles instead of just up and down.

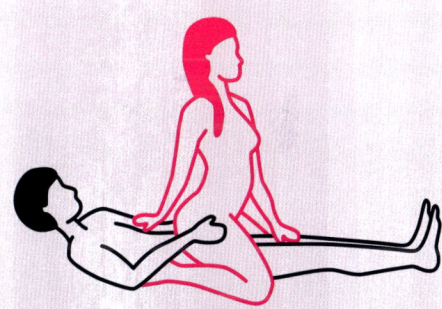

At some point, try arching your back, which allows his member to stimulate your G-spot.

And, since you have easy access to your clitoris, give yourself a hand if you need it.

Reverse cowgirl offers some benefits for your man as well.

For starters, he gets some sweet eye-candy with that amazing view of your butt. And you'll really turn him on if you play with his testicles as you grind him. Guys also get off on females taking charge, but that doesn't mean that you have to do all the work. If you start getting tired, have him wrap his hands around your hips to help with the thrusting. But make sure you don't bounce too hard or lean too far forward, or you could cause some serious damage to his manhood. And if he happens to slip out at any point, simply put him back in and keep going.

✱ RELATED TERMS:
fuck, positions, sexual intercourse

R

rimming

Also called a *rim job*, *tossed salad*, and *analingus*, *rimming* is oral sex involving mouth-to-anus contact. If you're ready to play around back there, start by putting your head near your partner's butt, spread his cheeks, and have at it with your lips and tongue. Try things like slow licks, kisses, fast tongue flicks, gentle swirls, or whatever else you are both into. A variation on doggy style, position-wise, will likely work best here.

As with anal sex, Tristan Taormino, a sex educator and author of *The Ultimate Guide to Anal Sex for Women*, notes that some people get self-conscious about cleanliness in the butt area. If you suspect rimming may happen at some point in an upcoming sex sesh, Taormino recommends taking a shower or bath beforehand, which is not bad advice for any sexual encounter, really. "Some people like to use an unscented baby wipe beforehand to make sure everything's superclean," she says. "For safer rimming, you can also use a dental dam or plastic wrap from the grocery store" to protect from STIs and other infections, she advises. A dental dam is the best way to protect against spreading infections, intestinal parasites, bacteria, and viruses.

Another position to test out is simply lying down. The receiver lies down on a bed with their hips and ass tilted up and a pillow under their pelvis. Then the giver crouches behind them on their knees, grabs the lover's hips for leverage, and leans into their butt.

RELATED TERMS: *anal, anal play, oral sex, rusty trombone, STI, tossed salad*

rough sex

Like BDSM, rough sex often involves pain-play (consensual, of course). Moves like spanking, hair-pulling, choking, tying someone up, and slapping can all be part of the fun for people who like their sex with a side of subversion. The appeal for most people is that it isn't romantic. It's animalistic, passionate, edgy, aggressive, and sometimes painful. If you have fantasies of being bent over a table while your lover pulls your hair and whispers sweet nothings that aren't so sweet, you might be someone who's into rough sex.

While there is no hard data that can tell us if the majority of people prefer rough sex, PornHub published an interesting study. According to their data, the porn category "rough sex" was viewed by women 106 percent more often than men. The search terms "hardcore" and "bondage" were also viewed at significantly higher rates than men. So what does it mean? Are women more interested in hardcore sex than men? According to PornHub, when it comes to watching it, yes. That being said, it doesn't necessarily mean she wants to have rough sex. Some people get turned on by watching certain kinds of porn that they don't actually want to re-enact in real life.

R

BECAUSE ROUGH SEX CAN GET A LITTLE … WELL … ROUGH, IT'S ESSENTIAL THAT BOTH PARTNERS ARE FULLY ON-BOARD. HERE ARE SOME THINGS TO KEEP IN MIND:

- **Discuss what you are comfortable with and what you want.** As in BDSM, you should absolutely sit down with your partner and discuss clearly and specifically what moves you dig and what is absolutely off the table. Any sex therapist will tell you that good communication leads to good sex. It can't be stressed enough—have a conversation with your partner beforehand about what kinds of moves, acts, or toys you want to experiment with.

- **Use a safe word.** This will make sure the agreed upon boundaries are respected during rough sex.

- **Start small.** If you are new to sexual experimentation, don't start with having your partner flog you with a spiked whip while screaming at you in a foreign language. Choose one activity or move that doesn't feel overwhelming to you; asking someone to spank your ass or tug on your hair are popular places to start.

- **Communicate throughout the experience.** If your partner is pulling your hair but it's not hard enough, tell them. Dirty talk is a great way to accomplish this without sounding like you're placing an order at the deli for that hard ass slap you'd like.

✸ RELATED TERMS:
anal, BDSM, consent, fuck, kink, sexual intercourse

rusty trombone

The act of performing a simultaneous rim job and hand job.

Like playing an actual instrument, this move requires coordination, agility, and rhythm. Similar to a 69, there is a lot happening at once, and it's easy to lose focus. It's like tapping your head and rubbing your belly except with more genitals. Although the move does exist in porn, it's not superpopular IRL. The term shows up most often in dirty jokes and raunchy comedies.

The way it works is as follows: A man with an erection stands with his legs slightly apart, while his partner kneels behind him, licking his anus (the *rusty* part) while simultaneously reaching around to the aforementioned erection to perform a hand job (the *trombone* part).

Alternately, a *rusty trumpet* is when the receiver of the act is a woman, and instead of receiving a hand job, she gets fingered (while also receiving oral butt stuff, because of the rustiness factor, of course).

RELATED TERMS:
anal, anal play, hand job, kink, oral sex, rimming, tossed salad

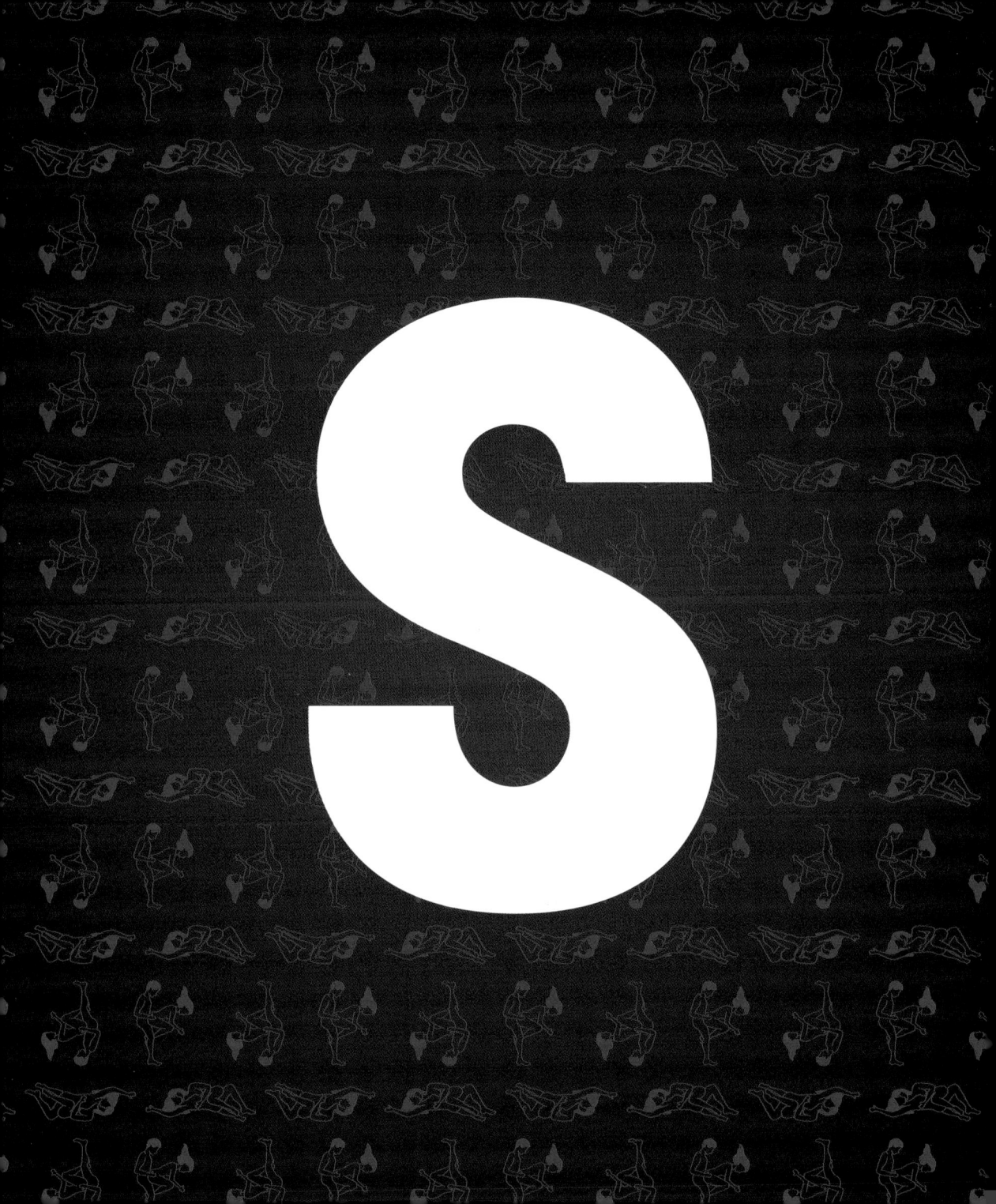

safe word

"When two (or more) people have a BDSM encounter together, generally they set a *safe word*—a word that anyone can say at any time to stop the action," explains Clarisse Thorn, author of *BDSM & Culture: 50 Shades of Stereotype* and *The S&M Feminist*. And just like picking the best password for your banking app, safe words are important for your security. Plus it ensures trust between partners.

HERE ARE A FEW THINGS THAT THORNE SUGGESTS TO HELP YOU GET STARTED:

- One commonly accepted phrase in the S&M community is actually *safe word*. (So unlike using *password* for your password, using *safe word* as your safe word is okay.) The appeal of it, says Thorne, is that if you get into partying at your local dungeon, future partners are likely to recognize your get-out-of-jail-free phrase when you scream it.

- *Red* is another safe word Thorne likes along with the other traffic-light colors used for checking in with your partner. "If I'm in the middle of an S&M encounter," explains Thorne, "I can say *red* and my partner will stop; I can then catch my breath and say *green*, which means *By God, keep going!* Or, if I'm a little uncertain about the territory but don't actually want my partner to stop—if I just want my partner to be a little bit cautious—then I can say *yellow* (and, of course, I can move to *green* if I become really psyched or shift to *red* if I really want my partner to stop)."

"The biggest moral of the story with safe words and check-ins," says Thorne, "is that consent does not only happen once. Consent is always happening, and can always be renegotiated or withdrawn."

RELATED TERMS: *BDSM, consent, kink, yes means yes*

> CONSENT IS ALWAYS HAPPENING, AND CAN ALWAYS BE RENEGOTIATED OR WITHDRAWN.

S

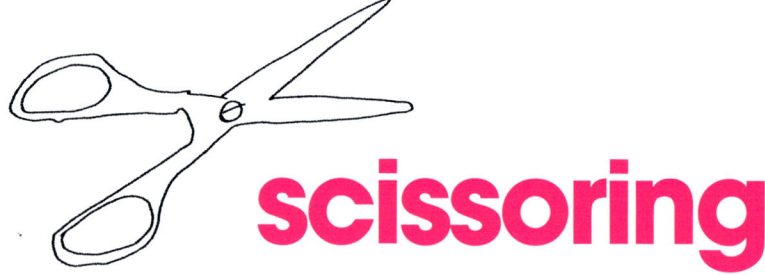

scissoring

Probably the most well-known lesbian sex position, it involves having one partner (let's call her Partner A) lie on her side while the other (Partner B) straddles one of Partner A's legs so their clits rub together. Then, well, they grind on, grind on.

If you want to try doing a modified scissor with your man, lie face-up on a desk or tabletop with your hips perched on the very edge. Raise your legs to an eye-popping 90-degree angle, then have your guy grab your ankles. He then extends his arms out to his sides, and as your legs are spread-eagle, he enters you while standing. Next, he starts alternately crossing and spreading your legs like scissors, opening and closing as he thrusts.

🌟 **RELATED TERMS:** *lesbian, lesbian sex, positions*

all about **semen** ...

Many things about the male human body are a mystery. Penises, why? Those tiny nipples, what?! But dip beneath the hairy surface of a man's skin, and even more mysteries await, hiding away in his male depths.

While usually contained safe and sound inside of the body, semen is a fluid most people eventually come into contact with but also do not know very much about. If it weren't for Samantha Jones calling attention to the phenomenon of funky spunk in the "Easy Come, Easy Go" episode of *Sex and the City* way back in 2000, women all over the world may have lived in quiet misery, forever perplexed by the unpleasantness of the male sex fluid.

To help educate the masses on the contents and, yes, healthy range of funkiness in semen, we spoke with a specialist about all things semen.

● How Semen Should Look

Aleece Fosnight, a urology physician assistant and sex counselor with the American Association of Sexuality Educators, Counselors, and Therapists (AASECT), explained that healthy semen should be a milky white or slightly grayish color. "Right after ejaculation, it's pretty thick," Fosnight said. "And twenty-five to thirty minutes later, it becomes clear and runny." The change in fluidity is to help aid in reproduction and thin out the cervical mucus to aid in the implantation of a fertilized egg.

● How Semen Should (Generally) Smell and Taste

Semen is a bodily fluid. Can you name any bodily fluids that smell like roses or taste like freshly baked cookies? No! There are none. So as a bodily fluid, you can expect semen to have a specific taste and

S

odor that isn't necessarily going to be lovely. Just to clear that right up.

The thing to note about semen is that it's a vehicle for delivering sperm through a vagina. So everything in it is meant to aid in that process. Semen is mostly made up of sperm, proteins, fructose (to help energize the sperm for transport), and seminal fluid. Fosnight said the typical pH of semen is around 7 to 8, or slightly alkaline. The vagina, on the other hand, has a pH between 3 to 5, or slightly acidic, so the alkaline nature of semen helps keep the sperm alive in an acidic vaginal environment. (Having fun yet?)

Because of its slightly alkaline pH, Fosnight said healthy semen should have an "ammonia or bleach-like kind of smell" and will taste a bit sweet (because of the fructose) and salty.

Fosnight clarified that semen left dormant for too long will start to develop a more concentrated taste or smell. Think of it like a stagnant body of water, collecting film and attracting flies. To keep semen from developing a stronger taste or odor—and also to promote prostate health—studies have found that ejaculating at least twice a week is beneficial to a man's health.

○ That Thing about Food Changing His Taste Is True

Let's go back to that old *Sex and the City* rerun, when Samantha made the spunky funk guy down a series of wheatgrass shots in an attempt to improve his semen flavor. According to Fosnight, that wasn't the smartest move.

Although there's been very little research done on the subject, healthcare professionals often hear anecdotally from patients that certain foods can slightly affect the taste of semen. While Fosnight said it's normal for fruits, which are high in sugar content, to change the taste of a person's semen, vegetables generally don't have much of an effect.

"Smoking can change the taste," Fosnight added. "It will have more of a bitter taste to it with smoking and with alcohol." So no one's saying you should avoid ingesting a mouthful of piping-hot semen after your partner's spent the night having too many drinks and then *whoops!* accidentally chain-smoking outside of the bar, but know that semen might taste especially bitter and, ahem, *spunky* after such an occasion.

4 myths about **semen**

Here are some facts you might want to know about this manly bodily fluid:

Myth #1: Sperm and semen are the same thing. The words are sometimes used interchangeably, but sperm and semen aren't the same. *Semen* is the whitish, sticky fluid released from the penis during ejaculation. It contains *sperm*, the male reproductive cells that can fertilize eggs if the sperm manage to make it from the cervix through the uterus to the fallopian tubes.

Myth #2: Sperm can only live inside the female body for one day. The American Pregnancy Association reports that sperm can live for up to five days, although it usually survives for more like three.

Myth #3: At birth, male bodies contain all the sperm cells they'll ever have. People with male genitalia aren't born with sperm—they start producing it at puberty, along with voice cracks, acne, and uneven upper-lip hair.

Myth #4: It's only polite to swallow your partner's semen. Um, no. Don't feel obligated to swallow. Some people love to and some hate it. Either option is fine. Live your life. (We've already established there is next to no protein in an average load, so if any guy tries to cite "health benefits" to persuade you, be sure to laugh.)

✸ **RELATED TERMS:**
balls, cum, cum shot, erection, ejaculation, genitalia, money shot, orgasm, penis

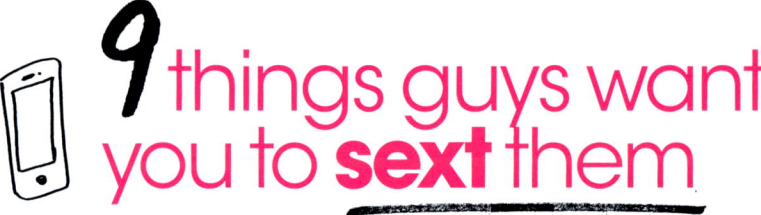

9 things guys want you to **sext** them

Boobs. If your mission is to sext, you can't go wrong with nudity from a guy's perspective. But remember that these images may stick around for a while. According to a survey by the Kinsey Institute at Indiana University, 23 percent of single adults reported sharing sexts they received with an average of more than three different friends.

Which is why **boobs that are covered** is the second-best—but still great—option. Some strategically placed objects(or your hands) can get him all riled up.

Detailed, descriptive messages about what you want to do to him later. And by *detailed* and *descriptive*, we mean you should try using lots of adjectives (like *wet* and *hard*) and talk in a lot of detail, as if you were explaining it to someone who's never had sex before. Also throw in something about you moaning and/or needing him.

A fantasy or sex dream you just had. Just letting him know you're turned on will turn him on, too. Horniness is like a yawn—it's supercontagious, even if you can't explain why.

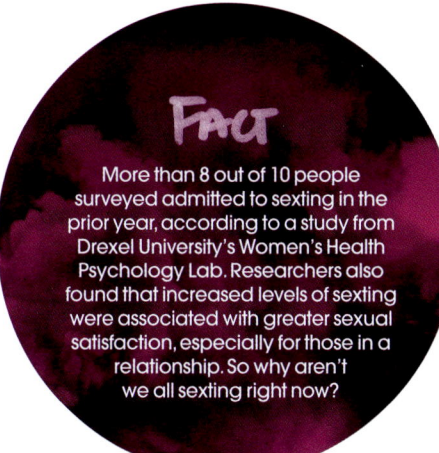

FACT
More than 8 out of 10 people surveyed admitted to sexting in the prior year, according to a study from Drexel University's Women's Health Psychology Lab. Researchers also found that increased levels of sexting were associated with greater sexual satisfaction, especially for those in a relationship. So why aren't we all sexting right now?

Tell him you just masturbated. It might sound kind of counterintuitive to let him know you just came without him, but the text "I just came thinking about you" will have him canceling all his plans, faking sick at work, and scrambling to get to your place.

Any text-only sext at an inappropriate time. Shoot him something sexy (not photos, just words) when you know he's in a meeting or out at a bar with his friends. He'll be all, "This feels so wrong." And it is. It's superwrong to have a boner while you're watching Jeremy from accounting walk everyone through a bunch of PowerPoint slides, but he won't mind.

A date-night plan (with sex included). The evening you planned includes that movie he wants to see and dinner at his favorite restaurant. Then you're going to take him home and tie him to the bed.

Send him a porn clip or pic, and let him know that's what you want to do with him later. Make sure the coast is clear (and he's not at work or in church or something) and then send him some "inspiration." Maybe it's a new position you want to try out, or some light S&M.

Anything but emojis. They just confuse things.

⭐ **RELATED TERMS:**
DILF, DTF, foreplay, GNOC, KOTL, MILF, sugarpic, TDTM, WSN

5 supereasy, not terrifying sex toys

Even if you consider yourself a sex-toy aficionado, with an array of Magic Wands and Rabbits buzzing away in your bedside table, you may not have had the nerve to bring out your faves when your guy is over. (That permahard XXL dildo can be a little intimidating for some dudes.) To get you two started here are our favorites to use with a partner.

1 A simple, palm-size clit vibrator. When you're first bringing sex toys into the mix, you need a reliable vibrator that your partner will be comfortable holding and using with you. If it has varying speeds and movements, all the better.

2 A vibrating cock ring. These are great because they're basically a hands-free vibrator for you during sex, plus it gives him a little jolt, too. There are many versions, from the most basic to some with impressive speed and strength levels.

3 A feather tickler. Yes, really. There's nothing more low-key beginner-sexy than this feathery friend. It's basically like an adult version of those spider-head massagers at the mall. The sensations are really subtle but also really powerful. Plus, it's just plain pretty.

4 A silky blindfold. Think of this as a beginner bondage. The silky-soft fabric won't make dipping your toe into BDSM scary, and the thrill of a little sensory deprivation is hot AF.

5 A partner-controlled vibrator. Technology is your friend when you have a vibrator that either one of you can remotely drive—even via a phone app from across the world.

❋ **RELATED TERMS:**
dildo, kink, masturbation, nipple clamps, vibrator

sexual intercourse

Traditionally, sexual intercourse is defined as the act of a man putting his penis into a woman's vagina. But if one thing is clear from the pages of this book, there are lots of different ways to have sex.

Now, if you've never had sex before, we'd caution you not to jump ahead to the advanced stuff right away. (Would a beginning surfer take on a 20-foot wave? You get the point.) The first time you have sex with someone is a deeply individual experience. "Sex" means different things and comes with different emotions from person to person (and from hookup to hookup, TBH). That said, there are a handful of insights that can make your first time having penetrative sex comfier, more communicative, and more pleasurable—all pretty universally great things for sex to be. Here are eight first-time pointers, with advice from sex therapist Vanessa Marin.

- **Being safe can actually relax you.** Nothing is more distracting than worrying about STIs and pregnancy during sex. Even if it feels awkward, it is so, so, so important to chat with your partner beforehand about what you'll do to protect yourselves. Use a condom even if you're on another form of birth control to protect you both from STIs, unless you are both monogamous with each other and STI-free (check out local clinics like Planned Parenthood for free/affordable testing).

- **Enthusiastic consent is a prerequisite for everything you do.** "Make sure you enthusiastically consent to each and every thing the two of

S

> YOU'RE MORE LIKELY TO ORGASM FROM ORAL SEX OR FINGERING," MARIN SAYS, "SO RESIST THE TEMPTATION TO THINK OF THESE ACTIVITIES AS THE THINGS YOU DO BEFORE MOVING ON TO THE 'MAIN EVENT.'

you do together," Marin says. "*Enthusiastic* is a key part of that sentence. Don't just go along with something; make sure you're excited about it." Remember that just because you start an activity—for example, intercourse—doesn't mean you have to finish or continue it: You have the right to pause or stop whatever it is. No. Matter. What. Same goes for your partner, of course. Check in with each other as things progress to make sure you're both enthusiastic about what you're doing.

- **Remember to breathe.** A big part of enjoying sex is focusing on the sensations you're feeling instead of, for example, your nervousness (which is totally common to feel your first time, even if you know you're ready to have sex). "Deep breathing is a fantastic way to let go of distracting thoughts," Marin points out. As you're taking those deep breaths, focus on how different parts of your body are feeling and how your partner's body feels against yours—not just the obvious part, but their fingers in your hair, hands on your hips, whatever it is.

- **Foreplay, foreplay, foreplay. Did we mention foreplay?** The more aroused you are, the better sex is likely to feel, so don't neglect foreplay—including oral sex, manual sex, and, yes, good old-fashioned kissing. "You're more likely to orgasm from oral sex or fingering," Marin says, "so resist the temptation to think of these activities as the things you do before moving on to the 'main event.'" Whether or not you do orgasm the first time you have sex, clitoral stimulation is the key to most women's pleasure, and vaginal intercourse doesn't usually provide very much of it.

TIP

Lube is your friend. A little bit can make sex so much more pleasurable. Another benefit of using a water- or silicone-based lube with a condom (avoid oil-based lube, which can degrade latex) is that less friction means the condom is less likely to tear.

- **Caring about your partner's pleasure matters more than your technique.** It's natural to worry that you won't be "good" in bed your first time, but trust: What matters most is that you are invested in how your partner feels and vice versa, and that you two are communicating about it. "A lot of people get anxious about sexual performance, but perhaps the best quality in a lover is enthusiasm," Marin says. "If you're genuinely enjoying pleasuring him, he'll notice it, and he'll have a lot more fun, too." Simple questions like "How does that feel?" and "Do you like it when I [fill in the blank]?" give your partner a chance to express appreciation for what you're doing or (gently) ask for something a little different.(As well as prompt them to ask you the same questions!)

- **Feedback is not the same as criticism, so don't hesitate to give it.** A common concern is that if you tell your partner something doesn't feel good—or something else would feel better—they'll feel attacked. But if they care about your pleasure, they'll be happy to hear how to help you feel it. In the moment, it can be hard to figure out what exactly you want, so it can be helpful to talk afterward about what you enjoyed, what you could do without, and what you'd like to try next time. And if you don't have an orgasm, don't feel pressured to pretend to have one. Think of orgasming not as your responsibility but as a fun goal to work toward with your partner(s), together.

- **Your partner's penis might not do everything the two of you want.** Whether premature ejaculation, a limp penis, or inability to orgasm strike, it doesn't mean something is wrong with your partner or you failed them somehow. Comfort with a new partner often takes time and communication, and that goes for both men and women.

- **Temper your expectations.** Movies and TV shows can sell us a pretty unrealistic vision of what having sex for the first time looks like. It's often perfectly choreographed, mood-lit, and romantic and ends in an implied simultaneous orgasm. As if. Don't expect fireworks the first time you have sex—sex is messy and human and flawed and often awkward, whether it's your first time or your thousandth. It's the practice and the exploration that make sex fun.

✱ **RELATED TERMS:** *consent, foreplay, fuck, lube, orgasm, penis, position, yes means yes*

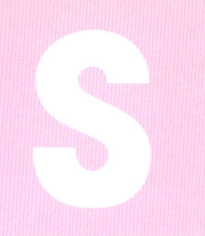

how to have **shower sex** that won't land you in the ER

Steamy air, cascading water, soapy naked bodies gliding against each other . . . Shower sex *sounds* incredibly erotic. In reality, the experience can be anything but. First, the close quarters and slick surfaces call for some pretty awkward maneuvering. "And there are physical dangers, like slipping and falling," warns sex coach Alicia Sinclair.

All that said, at *Cosmo*, we are undaunted by the carnal challenge, so we've come up with tips for safely pulling off a wet and wild session.

Get a grip. Holding on to your shower curtain as your partner takes you from behind can rip it down, and putting your foot on the slick edge of the tub for a better angle during face-to-face sex is asking for trouble. So be sure to make sure you have something secure to grab on to.

Bring a buddy. An inconspicuous vibrating loofah can help you lather up and act dirty at the same time. Have your partner work it all over your body, stopping at hot spots such as your nipples and clitoris for an X-rated thrill.

Light it up. Most bathroom lighting is harsh and unflattering—the opposite of mood setting. If you have a tub or a glass shower door, consider dimming the overheads and lining your countertop with scented candles for a sexy glow, suggests Sinclair.

Feel even wetter. Getting water in your lady parts can actually dry them out, making sex uncomfortable. Reach for a silicone lube to help keep the action slidey and glidey.

Rub-a-dub-dub each other. Give each other a scalp massage with shampoo. Then move on to full-body stroking with a lotion that won't mess with your pH levels.

Cushion the blow. A washcloth is not only an ideal accessory with which to rub each other down; it's also a great cushion for your knees. When you're going down on your partner or if you're doing it doggy style.

❋ **RELATED TERMS:** *bareback, doggy style, foreplay, fuck, lube, oral sex, penis, positions, quickie, sexual intercourse, vagina*

OOPS-PROOF POSITIONS.
Here are a few options to try:

The Bathing Booty:
Firmly plant your feet on the tub floor, and make sure they're secure. Then bend over at the waist and spread your legs so your guy can enter you from behind. He gets a stellar view, while you get plenty of G-spot feels.

The Edge of Glory:
Oral in the shower = an awesome adventure. Take turns sitting on the edge of the tub and pleasuring each other with your mouths. On your turn, switch up the pace of your tongue, twisting from long, slow licks to speedy circles.

The Stream Team:
Face your partner, lean back against the shower wall, and wrap one leg around his torso. Then have him enter you. If you have a handheld showerhead, aim the water at your clitoris while you swivel your hips back and forth.

S

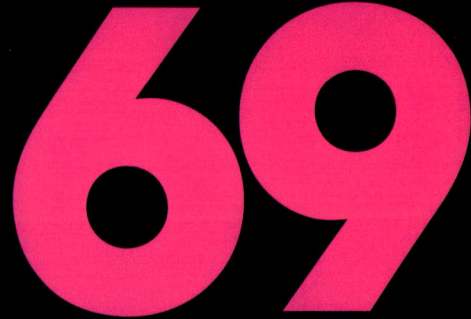

The act of two people simultaneously giving each other oral sex. To pull this off, one person must be inverted so each person can be positioned mouth-to-genitals. It's pretty obvious why it's called a 69—think of each partner's head as each respective bubbly part of the *6* and *9*. Once teen boys figure out what this means, they will forever snicker whenever they see the number. To be fair, everyone does.

This is one of those acts—kinda like shower sex—that might look better than it actually feels. It can be awkward, and, according to sex expert Calvert, it's easiest when people are similar heights. If one partner is 6 foot 5 inches and one is 5 foot 2 inches, it's logistically going to be a problem. If you're part of a male-female couple where height disparity can become an issue, Calvert advises, "It works better if the guy is on top, but you have to be comfortable with giving a fairly deep, rough blow job, which is what usually happens."

If you want to be in control, take the top. Have your partner lie on their back, then straddle their chest with your knees on either side, facing their feet. Then perform an upside-down blow job or cunnilingus, which will probably feel weird at first. Your genitals should be within reach of your partner's mouth. It can be difficult to concentrate on both giving and receiving pleasure at the same time, but if you can get everything to sync up, the position can be worth the effort.

✱ RELATED TERMS: *blow job, cunnilingus, fellatio, oral, orgasm, positions*

squirting

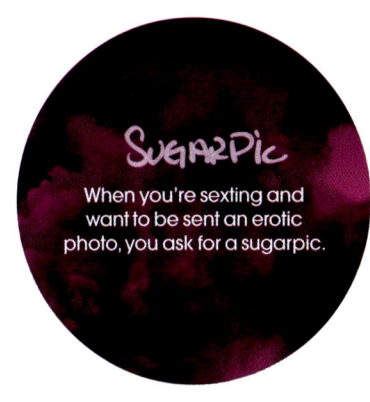

SUGARPIC
When you're sexting and want to be sent an erotic photo, you ask for a sugarpic.

This is when fluid comes jetting out of a woman's vagina, often accompanying orgasm. Sorta like having a Super Soaker® between your legs! However, not every woman can squirt, which makes it a topic of hot debate.

So what exactly is the fluid that comes gushing out of your vag? Is it pee, or something else? The answer: both, maybe. It could be that when some women squirt, they release a fluid from the Skene's glands, located on the upper wall of the vagina. This fluid is a combination of urine and prostate fluid. The weird thing is that it's also possible not every woman has Skene's glands, which further complicates the picture. The other theory is that squirting is orgasmic urinary incontinence, which is an involuntary release of the bladder during orgasm. Again, a lot more research is needed to know for sure.

Learning how to squirt is tricky. Sex expert Calvert says that if you want to squirt orgasmically, "get very comfortable with your Hitachi [Magic Wand®] and also get a G-spot toy." While there's no hard proof that you can teach yourself to squirt, there are definitely plenty of articles and Internet videos that try. Calvert notes that not all women can squirt and that when she does, only a few drops of liquid come out. Her advice? "I think focusing on 'I want to make this huge fountain out of my vagina' is unrealistic. It's much more about the sensation and the feeling and the orgasm, rather than how big a puddle you make."

To be clear, a lot of time, when you see squirting in porn, it's pee. "You can't tell [it's pee] unless the girl is really bad at her job and didn't drink enough water, so it's really yellow," says Calvert. "My personal experience is that I can't squirt on command. The porn makers are very practical about it. If you get hired to do a squirting scene, they don't really care what you're doing, if you're actually expressing the gland that creates the real squirt or if you're peeing." So it makes sense that sometimes squirting, like a lot of other things you see in porn, isn't real.

It's also a popular fetish, according to Calvert, which is why you see it a lot in porn—which may be what is driving the conversations about it. She theorizes that it's popular with men because they like to see tangible evidence (which is what happens when they orgasm) that a woman is coming.

RELATED TERMS: *fetish, orgasm, vagina, vibrator*

7 of your most STI questions, answered

Even if you had a sex-ed class in high school, odds are the section on STIs (sexually transmitted infections) was nothing more than a slideshow packed with icky images and a strong message to just never have sex. Or maybe you were lucky and had a great sex-ed program but need a refresher.

To continue your education, three gynecologists answered seven questions you might be too scared to ask out loud—but really shouldn't be.

Q: How often should you get tested if you're single and having sex with multiple partners?

In a perfect world, you should be tested before any sort of sexual activity with a new partner. And any new partners should be tested, too. Leah Millheiser, MD, an OB/GYN and director of the Female Sexual Medicine Program at Stanford University, said she sees a lot of female patients in her practice who get tested before their partners do, find out they don't have any STIs, and then never ask their partners to be tested. Making things even riskier for women, men are three times likelier than women to say they've never been tested at all.

Of course, the rule if you're single is to always, always, always use a condom, and be honest with partners and yourself about your screening history. If you feel it's time for a test, get a test. Don't be shy about asking any and all of your partners when they were last tested, either.

Q: Does one test cover all STIs out there?

There's actually no such thing as a blanket "STI test." What *is* a thing are tests that doctors use to screen for individual STIs. Chlamydia and gonorrhea can each be tested through a urine sample, a vaginal swab, or a swab inside the penis, while a blood sample or oral swab is needed to test for HIV and hepatitis. According to Jennifer Conti, MD, an OB/GYN, "A full STI screening includes both blood and urine tests and checks for HIV, syphilis, hepatitis B and C, chlamydia, and gonorrhea." But if you ever think you've been exposed to something not on that list—like herpes or crabs— you can talk to your doctor about testing for those individually at any time.

Q: Are STI tests always accurate?

No medical test is 100-percent accurate 100 percent of the time. Dr. Millheiser said it also depends on what type of test the lab is using and which STI you're testing for.

For example, herpes blood tests are often said to deliver false results. According to the CDC, false negatives are common shortly after contracting genital herpes, and false positives are common especially among people who have a low value of herpes antibodies. So the current guideline for herpes testing is to avoid routine screening and primarily test if or when someone is displaying symptoms.

"The most effective test [for herpes] is to actually do a swab on a lesion as soon as you see it," Dr. Millheiser said. "A blood test tells you if you have antibodies for herpes 1 or 2, but that doesn't necessarily mean you have genital herpes."

The testing method can also play a role in result accuracy. You can (and should) talk about all of the testing methods available with your physician. And, as always, see a doctor sooner rather than later if you have any symptoms—like discharge, itching, or bumps—that could be indicative of an STI.

Q: Where can I go for affordable testing for men and women who do not have health insurance?

Both Colleen Krajewski, MD—an OB/GYN and medical adviser to Bedsider, an educational site from the National Campaign to Prevent Teen and Unplanned Pregnancy—and Dr. Millheiser recommend Planned Parenthood, which is very much open to all genders, not just women. Dr. Millheiser also mentioned going to a free health clinic in your city. If you live in a rural area, check to see if your county has a local health department—most will offer free or low-price STI testing. The CDC also has a resource for finding free STI testing near you.

S

Q: Why do gynecologists not test for things like herpes and HIV unless you request testing?

This question is a bit complicated to answer. The only things on an "annual testing list" for women under twenty-five years old are gonorrhea and chlamydia, because they're the most at-risk for those two STIs due to the nature of their cervical cells at that age. HPV screening is done alongside a Pap smear, so every three to five years for women under sixty-five. HIV is screened every one to five years for people who are at an increased risk for contracting it, or at your request otherwise. And as mentioned before, herpes is only screened for upon request or when someone's displaying symptoms. Dr. Millheiser said that routine blood testing for genital herpes (or herpes simplex virus, HSV) just causes patients "undue anxiety," because the antibodies for HSV are common, even among people who've never had a lesion.

All that said, your specific routine screenings should be determined by you and your doctor. "Doctors will tailor all the tests to each specific patient based on preexisting conditions and prior diagnoses," Dr. Millheiser said. As with any medical procedures, you should never be afraid to ask your doctor which tests they're ordering, and feel free to ask questions about those tests and request others if you feel they're necessary.

Q: Is it necessary to get an STI test if you haven't changed partners since your last test?"

It's up to you. "I don't recommend it, but then I think patients are better at assessing their own risk than I am in terms of how much

> **FACT**
>
> A Cosmoplitan.com survey of 1,454 millennials supports this—47 percent of respondents said none of their past partners ever asked about STI test results before having sex.

they suspect something else going on," Dr. Krajewski said. In other words, if you suspect your partner isn't being totally monogamous or may be lying to you, talk to your doctor about being tested.

Or let's say you haven't had sex with anyone new but are worried you may have contracted something from your most recent partner even though you don't have any symptoms. STIs have incubation periods, and the incubation period for each one is different. Dr. Millheiser recommends seeing your doctor right away if you think you may have come into contact with an STI, and they can help you work out a testing plan. Dr. Millheiser gave the example of herpes. "If somebody has been exposed to herpes and had an infection but didn't show up to my office until a week after the lesion showed up,

the test may come back negative if it's already scabbed and healed over," Dr. Millheiser said. Herpes is a particularly good example because, again, it's known for delivering false results—so if a lesion pops up even though you haven't had any new partners, you should see your doctor and discuss testing.

The rule is to make an appointment with your doctor for testing the moment you suspect you've come into contact with an STI or think you're having STI symptoms, even if you haven't changed partners in a while. Your doctor will work out a plan for retesting from there.

Q: How do you tell your partner you have an STI?

Dr. Krajewski notes that one way to ease into an STI conversation is by saying something like, "Hey,

when was the last time you got tested, because I got tested [fill in the blank]." Opening the convo by talking about yourself makes it a little easier for your partner to talk about their own sexual history. It's a good way to make it feel less like a line of questioning and more like a casual conversation.

The most important thing, though, is to just be honest with each of your partners—the best way to avoid spreading STIs is regular testing, vigilant condom usage, and full disclosure. There's nothing shameful about having an STI, and any partner who makes you feel otherwise is almost certainly not worth your time.

★ **RELATED TERMS:**
condoms, consent, fuck, oral sex, safe word, sexual intercourse, yes means yes

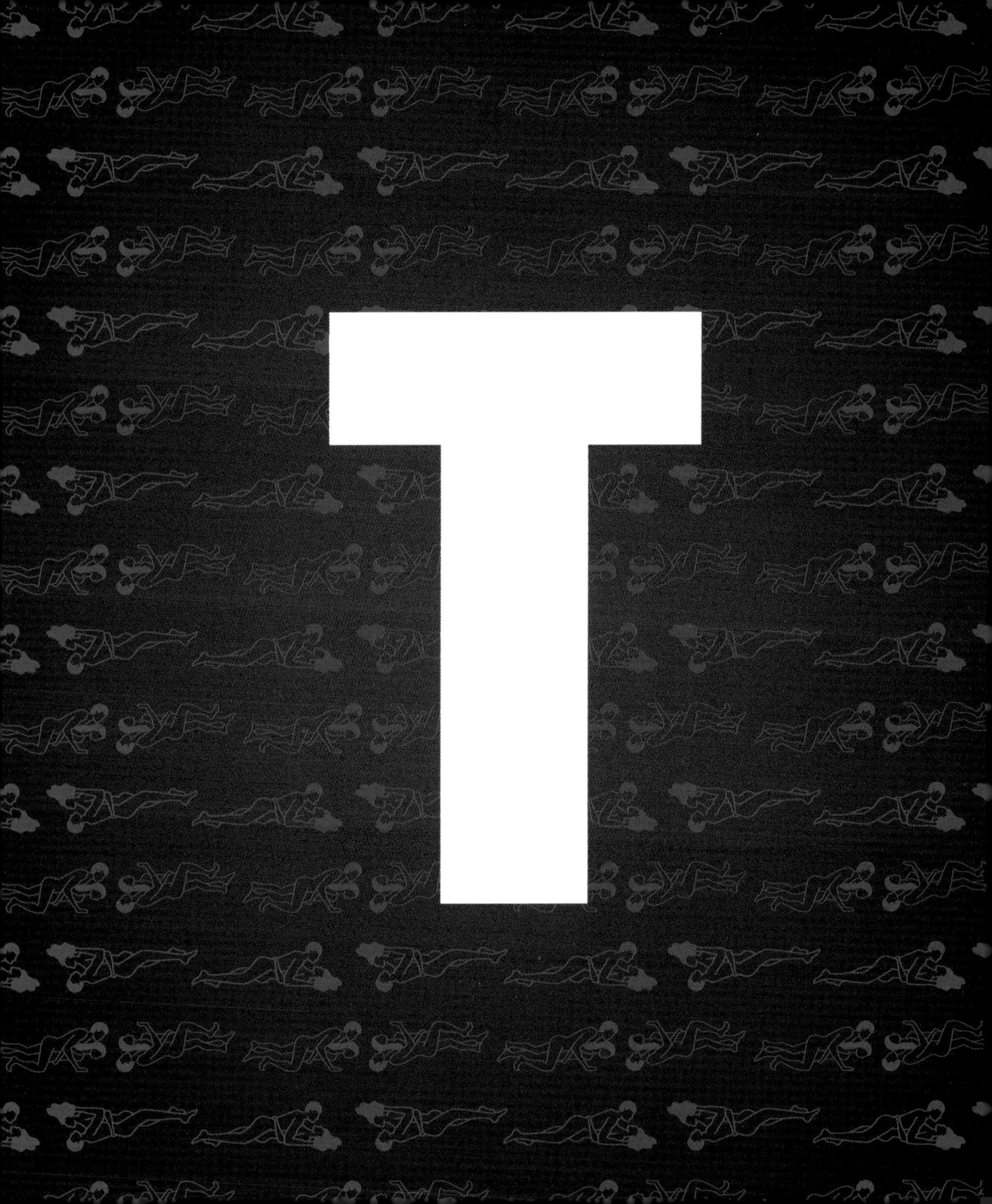

tantric sex

Ah, tantric sex... The words bring to mind images of yogis or superhot woo-woo celebs going at it for hours until, eventually, orgasming longer than even your most epic Netflix binge. But there are several myths about Tantra. Let's go back to clear things up.

Tantra began in India thousands of years ago, according to Dawn Cartwright, Tantra instructor and founder of the Chandra Bindu Tantra Institute. "It is an ancient path of meditation with roots in both Hindu and Tibetan Buddhist spirituality," she says. Although Tantra involves study, meditation, and breathwork, the aspect that people are usually most intrigued by is sexual practice because, duh, sex.

"Tantra views every facet of human experience, including sex, as potential for personal transformation and self-actualization," Cartwright explains. "For the tantric, life is a meditation. Every activity—eating, drinking, breathing, dancing, making love—can be entered into with awareness."

The idea behind tantric sex in the Hindu spiritual tradition is that when sex is practiced with awareness and connection, it is a way to achieve enlightenment. Tantric sex is focused on very slow intercourse, with an emphasis on synchronized breathing, touching, eye contact, and intimacy with your partner. Unlike regular sex, orgasm is not the goal; rather, prolonging orgasm and feeling a deep connection are the goals.

"Tantric practices focus on helping us to allow more of that natural energy to flow through us," adds Barbara Carrellas, author of *Urban Tantra: Sacred Sex for the Twenty-First Century*. Carrellas explains that although you can have a tantric quickie, "if you're being mindful and breathing more and you don't have a goal, but rather it's all a journey, you're going to slow down."

Slow sex benefits women more, anyway. Women generally take longer to get aroused than men, so tantric sex is actually more aligned with the feminine sexual response. A man taking his time with your entire body and not rushing you or pressuring you to climax? It could be worse.

T

TANTRA INVOLVES STUDY, MEDITATION, AND BREATHWORK, THE ASPECT THAT PEOPLE ARE USUALLY MOST INTRIGUED BY IS SEXUAL PRACTICE BECAUSE, DUH, SEX.

THERE'S NOT REALLY AN EXACT RECIPE FOR TANTRIC SEX, BUT THERE ARE A FEW TIPS:

- **Breathing:** Like in yoga, focusing on your breath helps to put you in the moment and make you more mindful, and it also moves energy within your body.

- **Slowing down:** Carrellas recommends the "three for thirty" approach. Meaning, if you would normally do thirty strokes of something, do only three in the same period of time. Tantra is obviously not for impatient people.

- **Eye gazing:** "In Tantra, we use eye gazing as the gateway into the soul," says Carrellas. "It puts you into a deep, altered state with someone."

- **Undulating:** Moving your body helps move that all-important energy around. Carrellas suggests "moving your pelvis and PC muscle as an energy pump, not just as a physical fuck muscle. Imagine the energy that's in your genitals moving up your spine into the rest of your body, over the top of your head, and onto your partner's body." Just don't laugh while you're imagining this.

- **Spooning:** Another tantric-inspired practice you can try is called the Daily Devotion, recommended by sex therapist and Tantra practitioner Jacqueline Hellyer. The way it works is you and your partner spoon every day in the morning with him lying directly behind you. He inserts his penis into you and keeps it there for five to ten minutes. Hellyer recommends "Just lying there, breathing together. No movement. Maybe the occasional vaginal squeeze. Feel what happens."

- **Wrapping:** If having nonmoving sex doesn't excite you, you can also experiment with the traditional tantric sex position *Yab-Yum*, which is supposed to encourage more intimacy and connection between partners. Yab-Yum is where a woman sits in the man's lap and wraps her legs around his waist, with both partner's arms around each other and both people's root chakras (or genitals) connected.

RELATED TERMS:
fuck, kama sutra, positions, sexual intercourse

TDTM

When you're texting your guy and want him to crank up the sexy, you might type TDTM, which stands for "talk dirty to me."

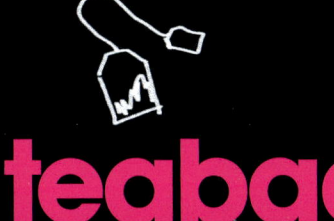

teabagging

If you love a steaming cup of chamomile and think we're about to share some secret about how it can improve your next sex session, sorry. This term has nothing to do with that. Rather, *teabagging* is the act of a man placing his scrotum into the mouth or onto the face or forehead of another person, usually while standing or kneeling over that person. (Think dipping a tea bag into a mug and you've got the visual.) According to Jessica Drake, sex educator and founder of the *Guide to Wicked Sex*, "I wouldn't say that I'm a fan of the term *teabagging*. It's more of a humiliation thing. To me, it sounds like a frat-boy joke."

While it has its roots in humor and humiliation, teabagging can also be an arousing act. Drake, however, would like it to be called *consensual ball play*, although we have to admit that's not quite as catchy.

If you want to give it a go, consider using your tongue to stimulate all parts of the scrotum, either as part of a blow job or on its own as foreplay. Drake also recommends "gentle suction." But since your partner typically has control over the lowering movement of his own scrotum, don't forget to make your voice heard with a safe word if it feels like too much all at once.

✳ **RELATED TERMS:**
balls, oral sex, safe word

T

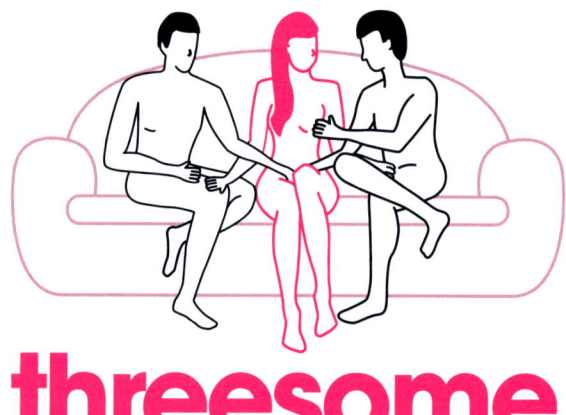

threesome

There's an old saying that "two's company and three's a crowd." But for some party people, three is just right when it comes to sex. The definition of *threesome*, according to *Webster's Dictionary*, is "a group of three persons or things" or "a golf match in which one person plays his or her ball against the ball of two others, playing each stroke alternately." It's fair to say that Mr. Webster probably did not have an active sex life.

According to Dr. Katherine Frank, author of *Plays Well in Groups: A Journey Through the World of Group Sex*, a threesome "refers to group sex between three people of any combination of sex or gender. All three may be single, or the situation may involve a couple inviting another man or woman into their bedroom. While the idea of a hetero couple looking for a so-called *unicorn*—a single woman willing to join the couple—is common, some couples extend an invitation to single men." The point is, a couple can invite someone of any gender to play. Threesomes, unlike golf, are nonexclusionary.

Before jumping into some tips on how to have a bangin' bang sesh with three people, you might be wondering where you even find people to do this with. Great question! Lucky for you, when it comes to kinky sex, the Internet provides many resources. Another option, if you prefer meeting people IRL, is going to a swingers' party. The swinger network is huge, with parties and get-togethers in almost every major and medium-size city. Get it, girl!

6 things to know before you try a **threesome**

Throples can be challenging to navigate, both emotionally and logistically. Dr. Frank has a few pointers for bringing another person into your bed:

Talk about boundaries and expectations beforehand, and be sure to check in afterward to make sure it went well and there are no hurt feelings.

Choose your third carefully, taking into account safety, whether you'll run into that person again, how attracted everyone is to one another, etc.

Treat all partners, but especially the newcomer, with respect. If you're a couple, you don't want to risk making a good friend feel like a third wheel. If you're a guy hoping to have a threesome with two women, don't assume they're bisexual or keep insisting that they kiss if they aren't.

If you're new to this, try doing it in a neutral location, like a hotel room. You don't want to be having sex with strangers in your bed and then accidentally catch a glimpse of that family Christmas photo across the room.

Communicate constantly with both people.

Embrace it all and don't expect a perfect experience.

RELATED TERMS: *consensual nonmonogamy, consent, fuck, kink, orgy, polyamory, positions, sexual intercourse*

tit fucking

Breast sex can be a sexy and natural move when you're slipping and sliding all over each other and find your breasts aligned with his D. But if you want to do it right, here are a few tips to know.

- **No boobs are too small—** although, admittedly, pushing them together may feel a bit painful. But the size doesn't matter to your guy. It's all about the visual.

- **There are two primary positions, depending on your cup size:**
1. Have him lie on his back and bend over him, pushing your breasts together. There's a reason that the most flattering boob-shot selfies are taken from that angle—for smaller-chested girls, thanks to the miracle of gravity, it gives you cleavage you may not have when you're on your back.
2. If you've got bigger breasts, you can lie on your back and have him crouch over you.

- **Don't rely on spit to keep your between-boob valley slick.** Saliva dries quickly and will only end in discomfort, so consider going with a silicon-based lube. It lasts the longest, and while it can irritate some women when used during penetrative sex, you don't have to worry about that this time.

- **If you want to free up your hands** for any variety of activities, use your upper arms to continue pushing your boobs together.

- **Oral is optional.** Considering that the head of his penis will be bobbing up and down toward your face for the next three to seven minutes, you could put your mouth on it. But that's totally your call.

- **Be aware that when he comes, you're at a prime angle** for a facial, so make sure to tell him where you want his cum to land.

❋ **RELATED TERMS:** *breasts, facial, fetish, kink, motorboating, pearl necklace*

tossed salad

Before you order one of these in bed, be sure you know what you're getting into. In the *Sexopedia* world, a *tossed salad* is oral sex involving mouth-to-anus contact. Wondering how it originated? Us, too! Unfortunately, there's no exact agreement on the history of the term in regard to sex.

RELATED TERMS: *anal, anal play, oral sex, rimming, rusty trombone*

T

transg

According to GLAAD, a LGBTQ media advocacy organization, *transgender* is "an umbrella term for people whose gender identity and/or gender expression differs from what is typically associated with the sex they were assigned at birth."

A transgender man is someone who was assigned female at birth but transitions to express a male gender identity. A transgender woman is someone who was assigned male at birth but transitions to express a female gender identity.

Pronouns are a huge part of the conversation when it comes to transgender people. According to the LGBT Resource Center at the University of Wisconsin, "When someone is referred to with the wrong pronoun, it can make them feel disrespected, invalidated, dismissed, alienated, or dysphoric (or, often, all of the above)."

> "WHEN SOMEONE IS REFERRED TO WITH THE WRONG PRONOUN, IT CAN MAKE THEM FEEL DISRESPECTED, INVALIDATED, DISMISSED, ALIENATED, OR DYSPHORIC (OR, OFTEN, ALL OF THE ABOVE.)"

ender

The struggle of being *misgendered* (aka being treated as a gender you don't identify with) can be extremely painful and traumatic. There is a psychological condition known as gender dysphoria, which, according to *Psychology Today*, is defined "by strong, persistent feelings of identification with the opposite gender and discomfort with one's own assigned sex that results in significant distress or impairment."

Many trans men and women suffer from gender dysphoria, due to the stress and trauma of not being accepted as who they are. This is a large part of the reason why attempted suicide rates among trans people are tragically high, at 41 percent according to National Transgender Discrimination Survey.

Being recognized for who you are is obviously a crucial part of healthy self-esteem, which is why everyone should address trans people with their preferred pronouns.

Courtney D'Allaird, coordinator for the Gender and Sexuality Resource Center at the University at Albany, uses the pronoun "they." They want the question, "What pronoun do you use?" to become as commonplace a question when meeting someone as "So what do you do for a living?"

But this philosophy certainly

T

doesn't apply to everyone. Some trans men and women fight hard to be treated and immediately recognized as a man or woman, and want very much to be addressed with a gender-specific pronoun such as *he* or *she*. So again, if you're not sure what someone would like to be called, follow their lead or politely ask.

According to GLAAD, one thing you should never ask, however, is if a transgender person has had surgery or is thinking about it. The condition of people's genitals, trans or not, is none of your business. Some trans people do opt for breast implants or genital reconstruction, some only take hormones, and some do none of the above.

In addition to fending off inappropriate questions regarding their genitals, trans people often have to deal with the concept of *passing*. To *pass* means to look like the gender with which you identify without people questioning it. D'Allaird notes, "Passing is, a lot of the time, about safety and being able to navigate your community or a public space without harassment or violence. It's also about acceptance."

But not every trans person puts an emphasis on passing. "For some people, it is a goal, especially when people start out in their gender journey; they're trying to be authentic and be accepted as such," says D'Allaird. "Then there are some people who do not seek to pass at all, because passing is just another form of oppression."

❋ **RELATED TERMS:**
androsexuality, asexuality, bisexuality, cisgender, gay, gender, genderqueer, heterosexuality/ homosexuality, lesbian, nonbinary, pansexuality, queer

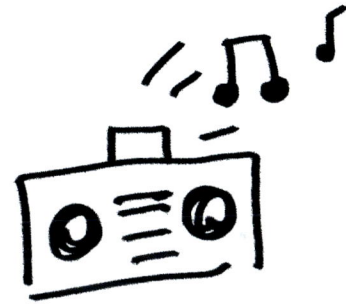

tune in tokyo

This is the act of twisting and fiddling with your partner's nipples as if they are radio knobs. This is sometimes purposeful and sometimes used to describe someone who is inexperienced and terrible at nipple play. Historians aren't positive why it invokes the capital of Japan specifically, other than that Tokyo's distant and would likely require a lot of effort to successfully reach. But the most popular reference to this "game" appeared in an infamous scene in the '80s movie *Girls Just Want To Have Fun*.

RELATED TERMS: *breasts, foreplay, kink, nipples*

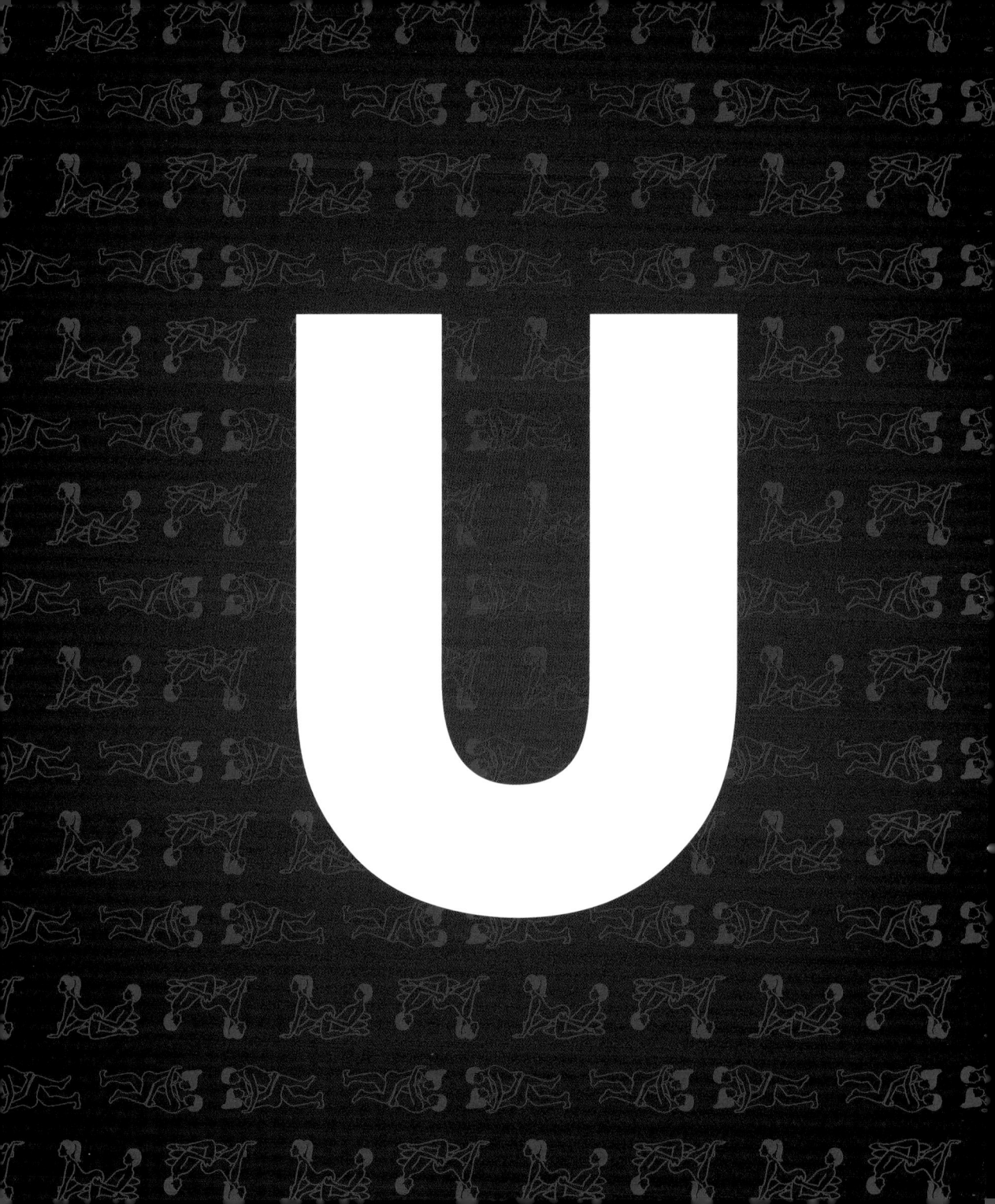

"ABOUT 61 PERCENT OF MEN WORLDWIDE ARE UNCIRCUMCISED ACCORDING TO A STUDY PUBLISHED IN *POPULATION HEALTH METRICS*.

uncircumcised

In an uncircumcised (or uncut) penis, the skin on the tip of the penis (foreskin) is left intact. And while all penises are unique, a natural one kind of looks like there is a turtleneck pulled up over its head.

If you've never encountered an uncircumcised penis, that's not unusual. In the US, most male infants still undergo the procedure. But what happens if you do land in bed with an uncut man? Here are a couple of things intact guys wish you knew about their au naturel appendages.

- **Uncircumcised penises may be more sensitive in general.** Even though there is much debate about this, start out being gentle with the head of his D and just check in with him about pressure and how he prefers you deal with his foreskin.

- **Beware of *phimosis*.** This is the inability to retract the foreskin covering the penis. While babies are almost never born with completely retractable foreskins, they usually develop them by the time they're teens if they're not circumcised. Possible causes of phimosis in adulthood include infection, scarring, and inflammation, and the condition is pretty rare—but if you're hooking up with someone who has it to any degree (or has other difficulty pulling back the foreskin), never force the foreskin back. Once again, ask a guy with an uncircumcised penis what he'd like you to do with it—and then have fun with it. You may even find that you prefer his all-natural penis.

✺ RELATED TERMS:
circumcision, penis

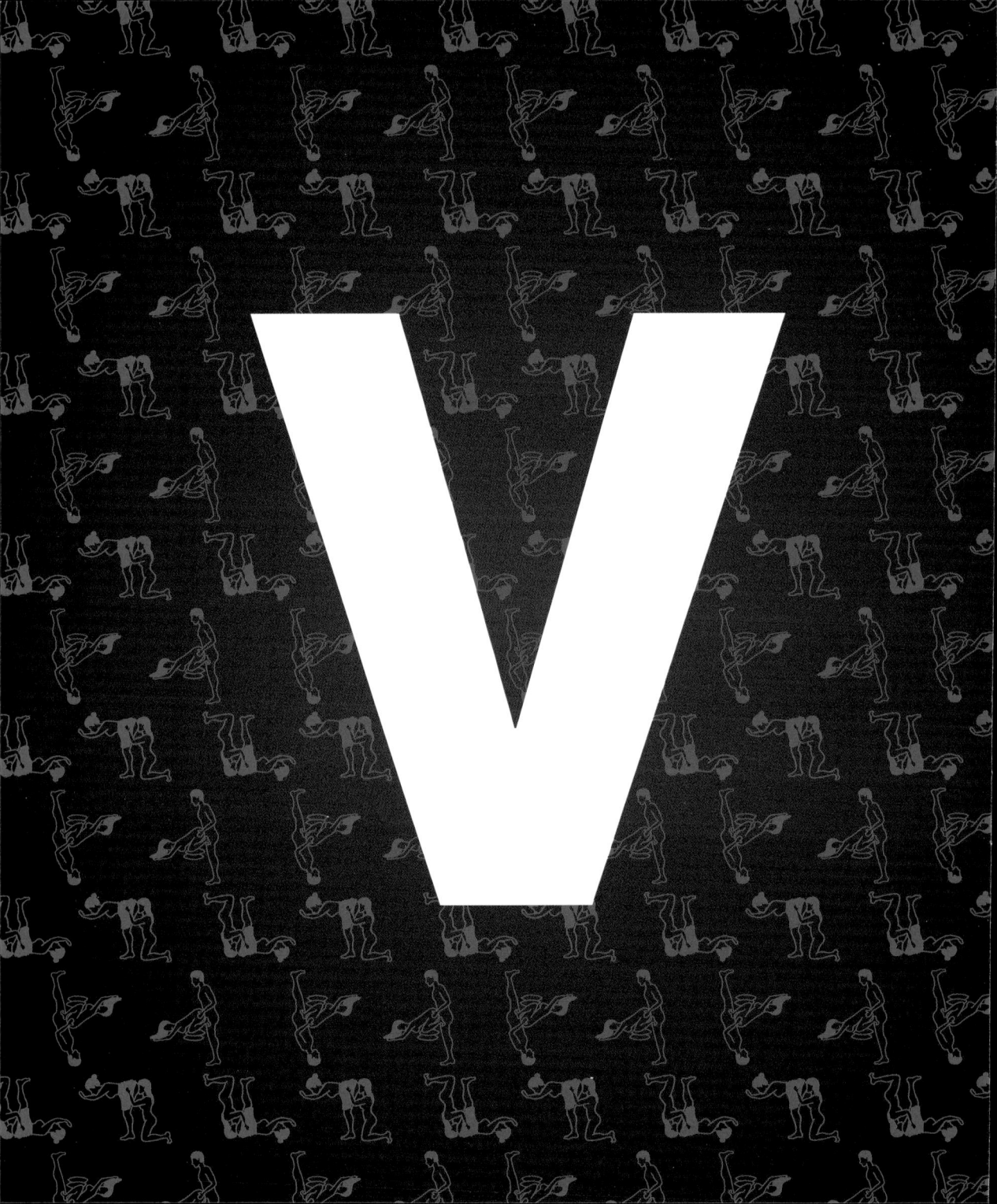

vagina

Just because you have a vagina (aka *vaj*, *box*, *coochie*, *hoo-hoo*, *honey pot*, *lady bits*, *muff*, *va-jay-jay*) doesn't mean you know about all the parts and structures that make up the female sexual and reproductive anatomy. It's okay if you aren't deeply familiar with each and every one—we got you, girl. OB/GYN Jessica Shepherd, MD, offers some insight to clear up some of the mystery around the female sexual anatomy and help create a society of wonderfully vulva-literate people.

- **No, what you see on the outside is NOT your vagina.** Despite popular use, *vagina* isn't a general word for the entire swath of bodily real estate below your hips and above your thighs. Vulva is the general term for the external parts of the female sexual anatomy. The vagina itself is a tube that connects the vulva to the cervix and uterus. It also serves as the birth canal during labor and is where menstrual blood flows from during a period.

- **The only part of the vagina you can actually see externally is the vaginal opening.** The opening is the center hole (of which you have three, counting the tiny opening of the urethra and the anus) that you can see on the vulva and is where you insert everything, from tampons and menstrual cups to fingers, toys, and penises.

- **You have two sets of labia.** They're called the *labia majora* (outer) and *labia minora* (inner). For more check out page 103.

V

- **And there's no rhyme or reason to which set of labia is bigger or smaller.** You might think *majora = bigger, minora = smaller*, but that is very much not the case. Labia actually come in a range of sizes, just like everything else about the human body. As Dr. Shepherd mentioned on page 104, a procedure called *labiaplasty* is available to people whose labia cause discomfort during sex or in their daily life.

- **The size of your clitoris has nothing to do with your level of sensitivity.** Some people have larger clits and others have smaller ones. It doesn't really matter either way when it comes to how sensitive you are.

- **The skin some people inaccurately refer to as the vagina is actually the *mons pubis*.** If you're looking at the whole thing straight on, the *mons pubis* is the mound of flesh directly above your vulva. It's what generally grows pubic hair once someone hits puberty.

- **Your cervix divides your uterus and vagina and is the thing you sometimes bump during sex.** As Planned Parenthood phrases it, the cervix is a little structure at the opening of your uterus that looks like "a doughnut with a tiny hole in the middle." This hole is where menstrual blood comes out and sperm goes in, and it dilates during childbirth. If you've ever had an

IUD placed, it's also what your doctor dilated to place the device.

- **Your uterus is where a fetus develops during pregnancy.** So it can also be called your womb, but truthfully, it feels creepy to refer to it that way unless there's a fetus in there. The uterus is pear-shaped and about the size of a closed fist.

- **When you're aroused, the uterus lifts up to elongate your vagina.** This is called *tenting* and is a really good fun fact to share if you're at a particular sort of party.

- **You have two ovaries, which is where all your eggs live.** Yes, it is true that you're born with all the eggs you'll ever have. Your ovaries are also responsible for producing the hormones estrogen, progesterone, and, yes, testosterone. Once puberty hits, they start to release an egg each month as part of the menstrual cycle.

- **Your ovaries don't switch off left and right with each menstrual cycle.** It's convenient to think that your left ovary releases an egg one month, then your right the next month, and so on and so forth. But as Dr. Shepherd explained, it's actually pretty arbitrary. She said that the ovary with the more developed egg, basically, is the one that's going to release it. So, theoretically, you could go three months on the left side. Bodies! So weird.

- **Your fallopian tubes connect the ovaries to your uterus.** And are basically like a big slide for your eggs. Sperm also travels through the fallopian tubes to get to the egg waiting in the ovary.

- **You probably still have your hymen, despite all the rumors.** Yes, even if you've had sex a million times, you probably still have your hymen. Dr. Shepherd said it doesn't tear and just go away, like all the girls in middle school said it would. What actually happens is the hymen stretches a bit, and that can cause a bit of bleeding the first time you have sex. So next time someone (rudely) says, "Yeah, you can totally tell if a girl is a virgin if she still has her hymen," please proudly say they are incorrect.

🌸 **RELATED TERMS:** *clitoris, G-spot, genitalia, labia, pubic hair, vulva*

V

vch piercing

A vertical clitoral-hood piercing is one that goes through the top of the clitoral hood and out the bottom.

RELATED TERMS: *clitoris, piercings*

---

vibrator

A vibrator (or vibe) is a sex toy that... wait for it... vibrates. While it's usually used externally on the clitoris or penis, it can also be used internally in the vagina or anus. Many women find using a vibrator during masturbation to be the easiest way to climax. According to Carol Queen, staff sexologist at online sex-toy store Good Vibrations, the clitoris and vulva contain nerve endings that are particularly responsive to the sensation of vibration.

It also can be fun to throw a vibrator in the mix when having sex with your partner for a little clit stimulation during penetration. Just a heads-up, if you're sleeping with a man, there's a possibility he might be a little ego-bruised when you suggest adding a vibrator to the party. Some dudes take it personally, like their penis isn't enough to get you off (Let's be real: Sometimes it isn't). Just assure him you love his special, unique, snowflake dick, but tell him you enjoy using toys to get off, too. If he's still being weird and doesn't want to do it, consider keeping the vibrator and ditching the boyfriend.

BUYING A VIBE

This may well be the most important decision a woman will

make in her adult life. Okay, maybe not. But it's a biggie. You can buy anything online if you're modest, but it's nice to go into a store where you can ask questions and actually touch and feel the products.

The most important thing to do when you're shopping at a sex-toy store is to find a salesperson you feel comfortable asking candid questions to. You want to be specific and let the salesperson know exactly what you're looking for. For example, if you prefer clitoral stimulation and don't want to put a toy inside you, tell them that! Feel free to ask what their favorite or most popular products are.

Once you choose your toy, make sure to ask about cleaning and sanitizing your product. Most rubber dildos and vibrators need to be washed with soap and water after every use, but each toy will have its own specific instructions.

You can find vibrators that range in strength from the superpowerful Hitachi Magic Wand to gentle bullet vibrators. Vibrators can be battery-powered, cordless, and rechargeable. The wand vibrator, which is smooth and shaped like a rocket (or a smooth dick, if you prefer to think of it that way) is a classic.

Queen says she often recommends a palm vibrator to newbies. Palm vibrators are shaped like a curved massage stone and fit over the vulva to provide external vibration to the clitoris and surrounding area. There are also some vibrators that are curved and meant to be inserted into the vagina. The point is, if you don't already own a vibrator, get on it. Literally, buy one and then sit on it. You're worth it.

There's some incorrect info about vibes that might spook you out of using them, so let's clear that up right now:

1. A vibrator will not make your clitoris less responsive to manual stimulation from your partner's hand, nor can you become dependent on one and unable to have an orgasm without it.

2. A common fear among men is that they can't live up to a vibrator, but that's not true. There's enough room for toys and boys in a woman's life, so no need to choose, says Sofia Jawed-Wessel, a sex researcher and assistant professor at the University of Nebraska at Omaha.

RELATED TERMS:
masturbation, sex toys

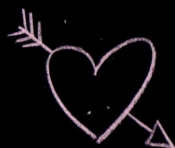
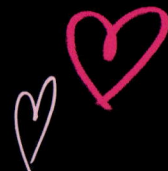

virgin

A virgin is someone who hasn't yet had sex. And, to be clear: There is nothing, and we mean absolutely nothing, wrong with being a virgin—whatever age you are.

Sure, some people are judgy about all kinds of sexual choices, but that's not us! If you are hanging onto your virginity, don't feel you have to hide it or be ashamed—there's plenty of time for you to have plenty of sex with the right person/people in future, if that's what you want!

RELATED TERMS: *fuck, penis, sexual intercourse, vagina*

5 things you need to know about your **vulva**

You thought you knew all there was to know about vulvas? HA, think again.

Not to troll here, but a lot of people refer to the whole crotch area as the vagina, which is inaccurate. According to the American College of Obstetricians and Gynecologists, *vulva* is the general term for the "external female genital area."

It's got a few parts. The vulva encompasses both sets of labia (majora and minora), the head of the clitoris, the opening of the urethra, and the vaginal opening. It can vary in color. The skin covering the vulva isn't always the same exact shade as the skin covering the rest of the body—it's totally normal for skin down there to be slightly lighter or darker than the rest of your bod.

Some STIs have vulvar symptoms. Like genital herpes (or herpes simplex virus, HSV), which produces visible lesions on and around the vulva during an outbreak. These lesions look like tiny red sores and usually appear in little clusters. HSV is most commonly spread during an outbreak, but can be spread at any time (really) by someone with the virus (which is very common). If you notice sores, your doctor can most accurately test for HSV by swabbing one.

Other STIs can be spread through vulva contact, like *trichomoniasis*, which is technically a parasite that's easily spread through sex, sex-toy sharing, and vulva-to-vulva contact. Planned Parenthood says 7 out of 10 people with trich never show any symptoms at all, but when present, they're similar to symptoms of vaginitis (green, yellow, gray, or bad-smelling discharge; blood in vaginal discharge; itching and irritation near the vagina; pain during sex; and painful urination).

It needs very little special care. Aside from the things everyone should be doing to just generally stay healthy—regular STI tests, proper condom usage, regular showers—your vulva doesn't need a whole lot of extra attention. In fact, most irritation of the vulva is caused by giving it too much attention through things like vigorous scrubbing, scented products, or constant hair removal. Leave the vulva alone, and it will leave you alone back.

✱ **RELATED TERMS:** *clitoris, G-spot, genitalia, hair removal, labia, pubic hair, vagina*

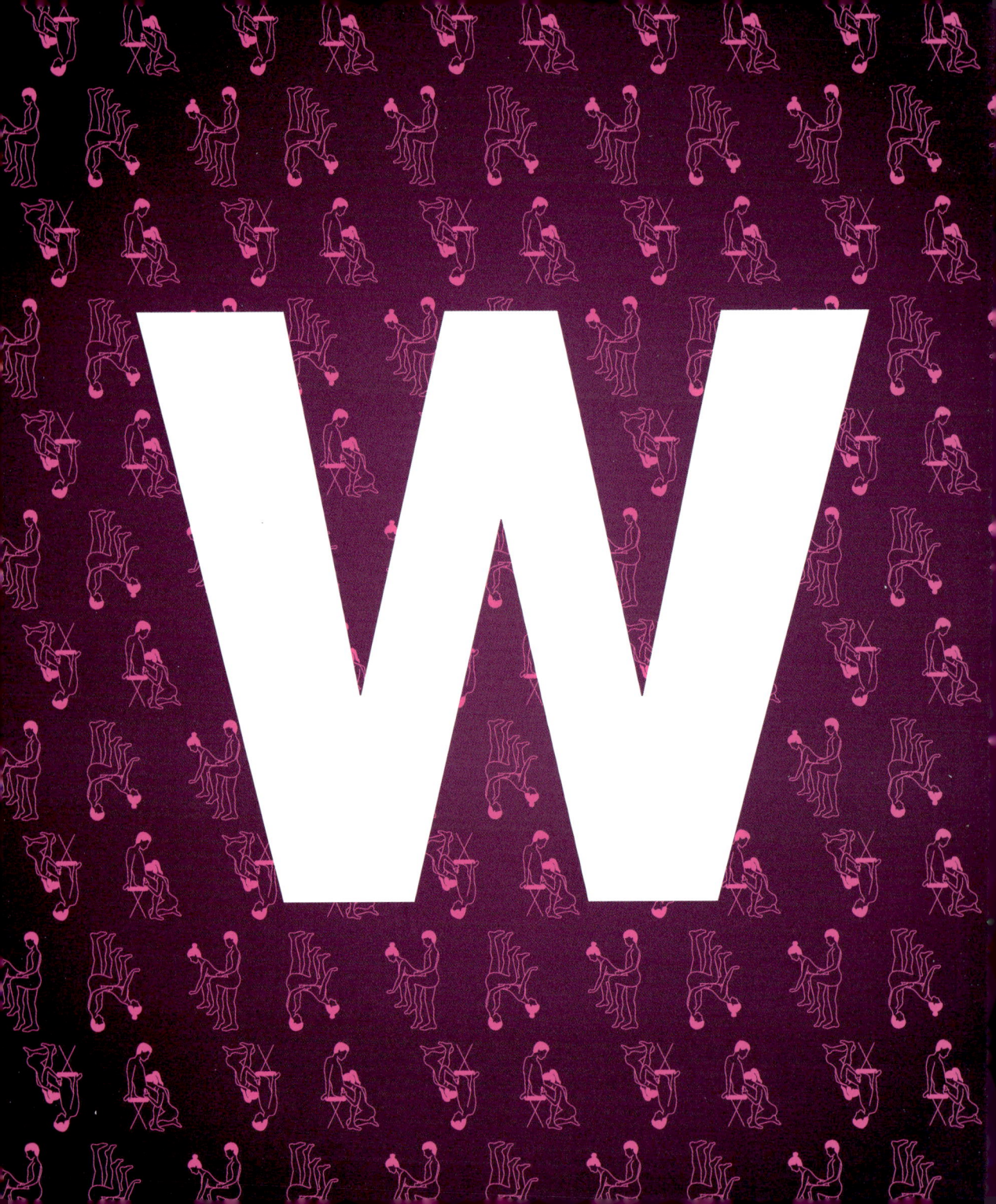

wank

Jerking off. Slapping the salami. Spanking the monkey. Rubbing one out. Apparently, men really like nicknames for masturbation, and *wank* is yet another one. A British one, to be specific. According to the *Oxford Living Dictionary*, the "vulgar slang" term was first used in the 1940s. And the term *wanker* is generally used to mean "a contemptible person."

RELATED TERMS: *jerking off, masturbation, orgasm, penis*

W

watersports

This isn't about paddle boarding or yachting with your crew but an activity some people find fun: peeing on a partner.

While there are other terms for this fetish—hello, *golden shower* and *piss play*—officially it's called *urophilia*, which can be found in the dictionary of words no one ever uses. (Also in that dictionary, btw, is *corophilia*, meaning an abnormal interest and pleasure in feces and defecation.) Ahem, moving on.

According to SexInfo Online, which is affiliated with the University of California, Santa Barbara, urophilia is "a sexual variation where people derive pleasure from urine or urination. The arousal is associated with smelling, feeling, or tasting urine, as well as urinating on someone or being urinated on by someone else. Sometimes, the pleasure derives from the physical urine (i.e., the warmth and the smell). Other times the person associates the urine and urination with intimacy, closeness, and trust. Urination can play a role in sadomasochistic activities, where the sadist will demonstrate dominance by urinating on the masochist. Some women find that their orgasms are more intense and pleasurable when they have a full bladder, or when they urinate during orgasm."

RELATED TERMS: *BDSM, fetish, golden shower, squirting*

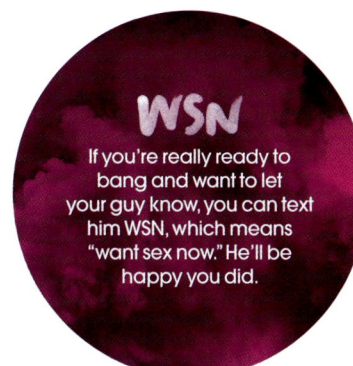

WSN
If you're really ready to bang and want to let your guy know, you can text him WSN, which means "want sex now." He'll be happy you did.

wet dreams

Nocturnal emissions—or spontaneous ejaculation at night—can happen to boys during adolescence and even adulthood. But it turns out that women may have their own version of sleepy-time delight, according to Kinsey Confidential from the Kinsey Institute for Research in Sex, Gender, and Reproduction. Scientists have found that during REM sleep, blood flow to the genitals increases—sometimes just a little bit and other times as much as it does when women masturbate or watch erotic films. This may explain why many women occasionally wake up from a deep sleep feeling aroused or having just had an orgasm.

✱ **RELATED TERMS:** *erection, nocturnal emission, orgasm*

---

withdrawal

While you shouldn't necessarily believe a dude when he says, "Don't worry, I'll pull out before I come," some people do use a withdrawal-method-and-condom-combo as a form of birth control. But be sure to talk with your doctor about all your birth control options. And whatever you do, make sure you consider STIs and pregnancy risks before choosing how to protect yourself during sex.

✱ **RELATED TERMS:** *condoms, fuck, sexual intercourse, STI*

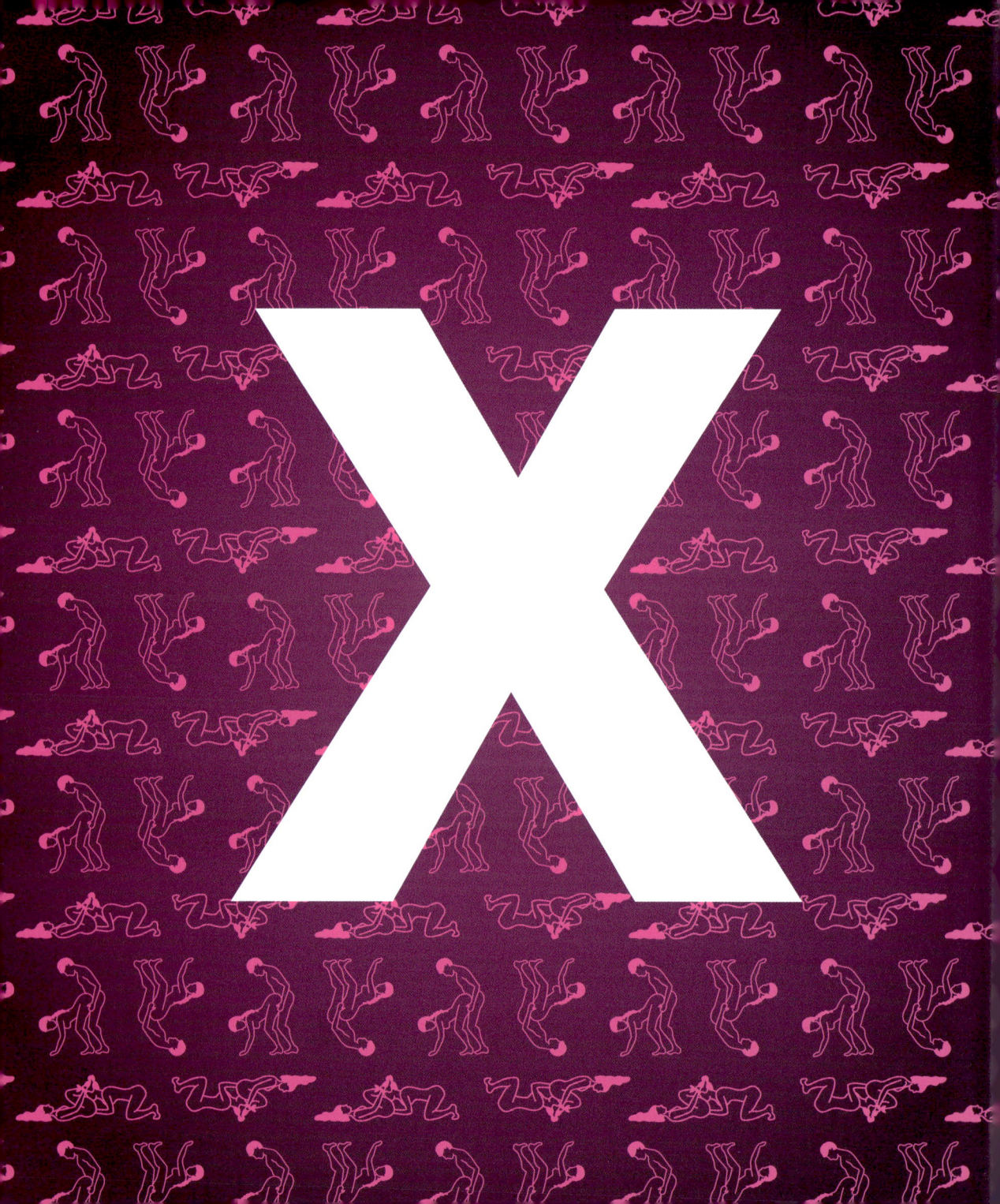

x-rated

When the Motion Picture Association of America (MPAA) introduced the X rating in 1968, it was meant to denote a film suitable for adults only—not necessarily because it had sexual content. However, in the film world, it's become synonymous with porn, explains documentary filmmaker Tony Comstock in *The Atlantic*. A triple X rating (XXX) isn't actually an official designation but simply a marketing ploy, explains Comstock. One film used it with the tagline SO ADULT, ONE X ISN'T ENOUGH!

Outside of the motion picture world, X-rated definitely refers to something that is sexually spicy, as in "My Insta feed is practically X-rated."

RELATED TERMS: *fuck, sexual intercourse*

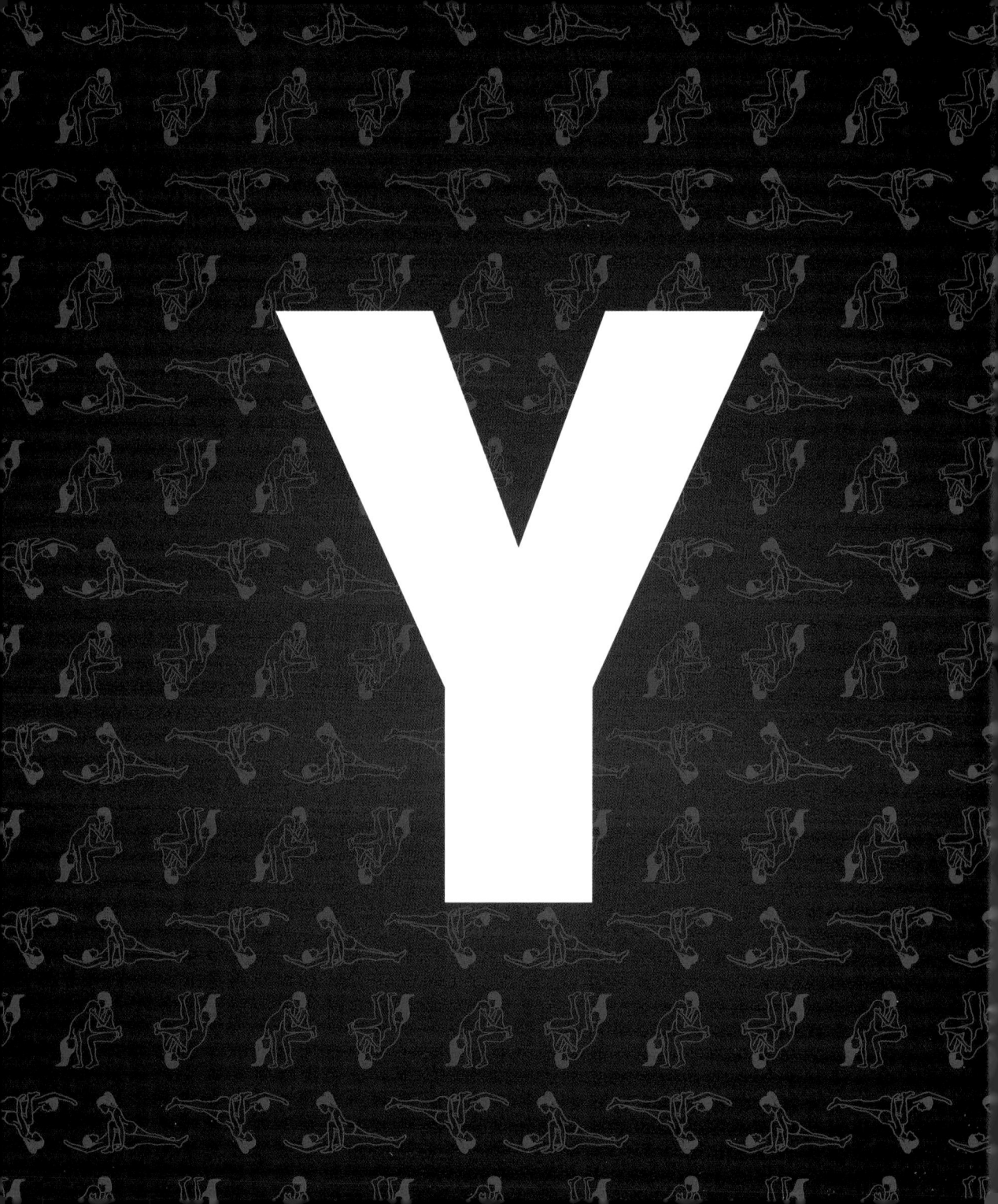

yes means yes

We are all about consent, and so is "yes means yes." In the past, "no means no" was the go-to language around sexual assault prevention, but it put the burden on the victim to resist and say no. "Yes means yes" flips the script and has been adopted as the standard at many universities across the country. According to the End Rape on Campus (EROC) organization, "In 2014, California garnered widespread attention when Governor Brown signed the nation's first affirmative consent standard for colleges to use in campus sexual-assault cases. The law established that consent is a voluntary, affirmative, conscious agreement to engage in sexual activity, that it can be revoked at any time, that a previous relationship does not constitute consent, and that coercion or threat of force can also not be used to establish consent. Affirmative consent can be given either verbally or nonverbally. Additionally, the law clarified that a person who is incapacitated by drugs or alcohol, or is either not awake or [not] fully awake, is also incapable of giving consent."

RELATED TERMS: *consent, fuck, safe word, sexual intercourse*

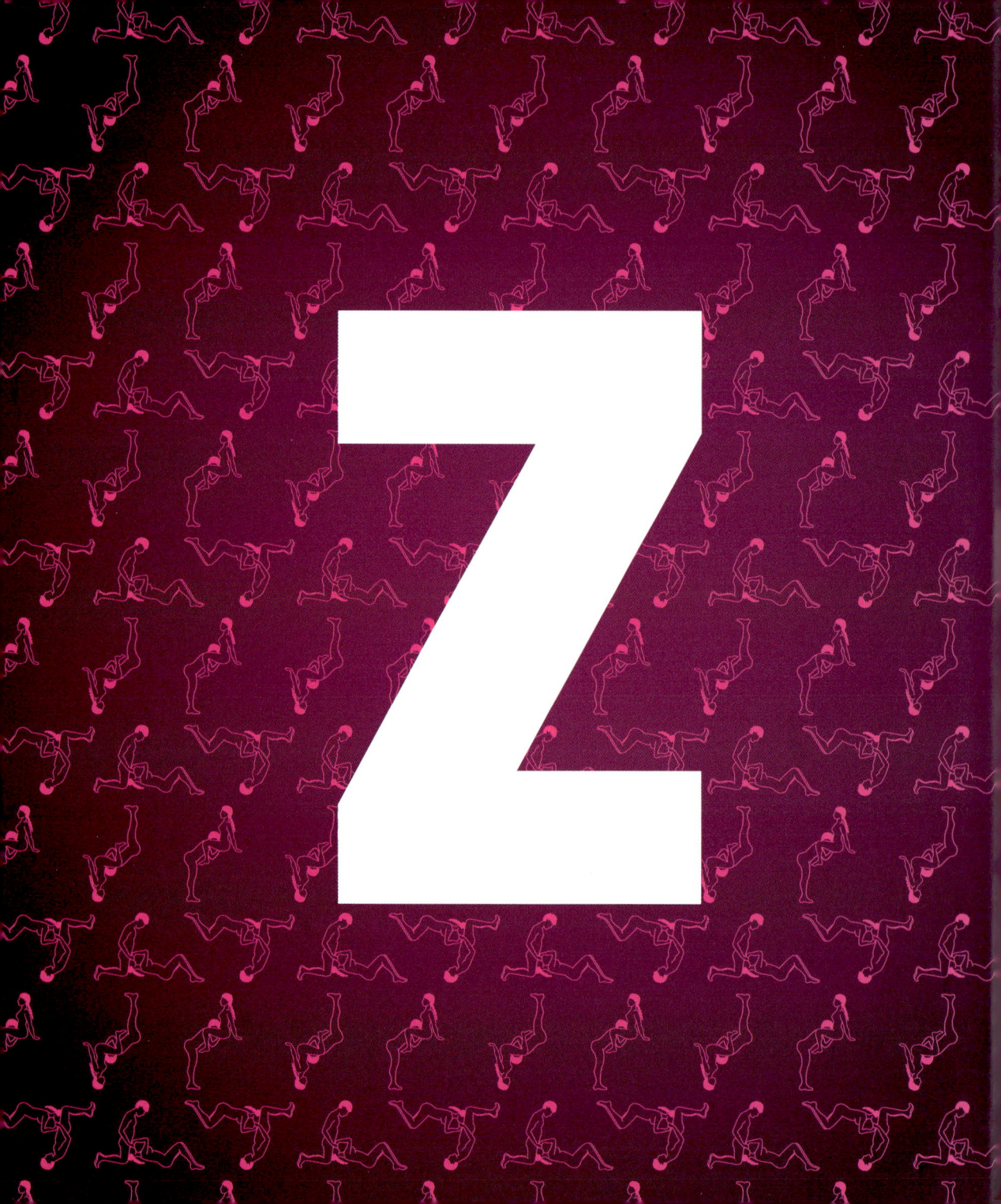

z-job

Giving a blow job to your guy while he's still catching some zzzs is called a Z-job. Though if this is the first time you're thinking of trying it out, you should confirm in advance that your partner is okay with you giving him a wakeup call via his morning wood. Consent is everything.

WANT TO UP YOUR BLOW JOB GAME? HERE ARE A FEW THINGS TO TRY WITH YOUR GUY:

- **Focus your mouth on the head while lightly gripping his shaft with both hands,** letting them follow as you move your head up and down, massaging with your tongue. Combining moves will keep you both from getting bored.

- **Use your tongue to stimulate other nonpenis parts** of your partner, like his inner thigh or right above his crotch. Your mouth in that general neighborhood will heighten all his nerves, making the actual BJ-sitch all the more exciting.

- **Cup one hand around the base of his penis and lightly squeeze,** using the other hand to assist your mouth as you stimulate his head and upper-shaft.

- **Keeping your tongue flat, start at the underside of his balls** and lick your way up to the tip-top of his head, like how you'd lick an ice cream cone. On the way up, you'll hit pretty much every erogenous zone down there.

- **Balls! They're down there, too.** You can do things with them, should you so choose, like gently licking or sucking on them as you're holding his shaft. Or, don't!

- **Swirl your tongue around the underside of the head of his penis, like how you'd lick a lollipop.** This activates the supersensitive nerve endings in his *frenulum*—the V-notch on the underside of his head, which houses the most sensitive skin on his entire body. For a variation, try flicking that zone with the tip of your tongue.

- **This is super simple, but try using just one hand for stability** during a blow job and touching your clitoris at the same time with the other, because there's no reason this should be all about him.

✷ RELATED TERMS:
balls, blow job, consent, fellatio, foreplay, morning wood, oral sex, penis, yes means yes

z

zelophobia

Nobody likes a jealous type... but if a person is really over-the-top, like cray-cray freaked out by jealous peeps, they probably suffer from zelophobia. So what if your bae is zelophobic? Here are a few ways to deal:

1 Recognize when you're being a jealous weirdo. A lot of the time when you feel jealous, you'll start little arguments or say passive-aggressive things rather than talk about what's actually bothering you. If you can acknowledge "Oh, I'm really jealous right now because he was talking to a girl at the bar last night and it made me feel weird," that's an important first step.

2 Look at your relationship from the perspective of one of your friends. If you were your friend and you heard about your situation, how would you react? Would you be freaked out, or would you think it sounded totally normal and probably fine? Putting some distance between you and your relationship always helps you to see things more clearly.

3 Focus on how great your relationship actually is. So you saw what looked like your boyfriend flirting with one of his female friends. Okay. But keep in mind, you two have an entire history and probably have a pretty unmatched closeness. Everyone flirts, sometimes without being conscious of it. It doesn't always mean they want to act on it.

> "YOUR CURRENT PARTNER HAS NO TIES TO ANYTHING THAT CAME BEFORE, SO PUTTING THEM IN THE SAME LEAGUE AS PEOPLE WHO HURT YOU OR THE PEOPLE YOU LOVED IN THE PAST ISN'T FAIR TO EITHER OF YOU.

4 Figure out if there's any underlying reason why you're jealous. Sometimes, when we're having feelings of jealousy about a partner, it's actually just because we're pissed at them for something else. Maybe they forgot a birthday or haven't been that supportive lately, and instead of just talking to them about it, it's easier to suddenly become suspicious of everything they're doing. That might not be totally conscious, but it happens.

5 Let go of any old relationship garbage that has nothing to do with your guy. Maybe you're worried about him cheating because your ex-boyfriend cheated on you or your dad cheated on your mom, but that situation isn't the same one you're in now (hopefully). Your current partner has no ties to anything that came before, so putting them in the same league as people who hurt you or the people you loved in the past isn't fair to either of you.

6 Recognize just how amazing you are. A lot of the time when we're jealous, it's because some part of us believes that we're unlovable and that our partner could do better, so obviously they would and will. But it just isn't true. You, right now, with all your flaws and shortcomings and struggles, are super-crazy lovable and worthy of having a committed partner, which is why you currently have one! Don't let some pointless belief that you're not as good as the hot girl he talked to at lunch mess with your head. 'Cause honestly, you rock, girl. Seriously.

RELATED TERMS: *allorgasmia, anorgasmia, erotophilic/erotophobic, ithyphallophobia*

HEARST BOOKS

An Imprint of Sterling Publishing Co., Inc.
1166 Avenue of the Americas
New York, NY 10036

HEARST BOOKS and COSMOPOLITAN are registered trademarks and the distinctive Hearst Books and Cosmopolitan logos are trademarks of Hearst Communications, Inc.

© 2019 Hearst Communications, Inc.

All rights reserved. No part of this publication may be reproduced, stored in a retrieval system, or transmitted in any form or by any means (including electronic, mechanical, photocopying, recording, or otherwise) without prior written permission from the publisher.

ISBN 978-1-61837-276-5

Hearst Communications, Inc. has made every effort to ensure that all information in this publication is accurate. However, due to differing conditions, tools, and individual skills, Hearst Communications, Inc. cannot be responsible for any injuries, losses, and/or damages that may result from the use of any information in this publication.

Distributed in Canada by Sterling Publishing, Inc.
c/o Canadian Manda Group, 664 Annette Street
Toronto, Ontario M6S 2C8, Canada
Distributed in the United Kingdom by GMC Distribution Services
Castle Place, 166 High Street, Lewes, East Sussex BN7 1XU, England
Distributed in Australia by NewSouth Books
University of New South Wales, Sydney, NSW 2052, Australia

For information about custom editions, special sales, and premium and corporate purchases, please contact Sterling Special Sales at 800-805-5489 or specialsales@sterlingpublishing.com.

Manufactured in China

2 4 6 8 10 9 7 5 3 1

sterlingpublishing.com
cosmopolitan.com

Cover and interior design by Kristen Male
Doodle illustrations by *Cosmopolitan*
Positions illustrations by Katie Buckleitner